Maroua Garma
Adel Bouguezzi
Habib Hamdi

Management of sinus membrane perforations during sinus lift surgery

Maroua Garma
Adel Bouguezzi
Habib Hamdi

Management of sinus membrane perforations during sinus lift surgery

ScienciaScripts

Imprint

Any brand names and product names mentioned in this book are subject to trademark, brand or patent protection and are trademarks or registered trademarks of their respective holders. The use of brand names, product names, common names, trade names, product descriptions etc. even without a particular marking in this work is in no way to be construed to mean that such names may be regarded as unrestricted in respect of trademark and brand protection legislation and could thus be used by anyone.

Cover image: www.ingimage.com

This book is a translation from the original published under ISBN 978-620-6-72585-5.

Publisher:
Sciencia Scripts
is a trademark of
Dodo Books Indian Ocean Ltd. and OmniScriptum S.R.L publishing group

120 High Road, East Finchley, London, N2 9ED, United Kingdom
Str. Armeneasca 28/1, office 1, Chisinau MD-2012, Republic of Moldova, Europe
Printed at: see last page
ISBN: 978-620-8-22060-0

Contents

Introduction

The sinus lift, or sinus elevation, is a sophisticated surgical procedure used in dental implantology to compensate for insufficient bone in the upper jaw. This procedure makes it possible to increase the height of the bone in this region in order to create an environment conducive to the placement of dental implants, while respecting the noble anatomical structure of this area, which is the maxillary sinus. However, this technique is not without its challenges, and one of the major obstacles lies in the management of perforations of the sinus membrane.

The delicate and fragile sinus membrane can be unintentionally perforated during sinus lift surgery, exposing the surgical site to sinus fluids and increasing the risk of post-operative complications. Proper management of these perforations is crucial to the long-term success of the procedure and the preservation of the patient's oral health.

Various methods are proposed for dealing with sinus membrane perforation.

The aim of this book is to detail the different techniques for managing the sinus membrane during sinus lift, while discussing a clinical case and referring to an in-depth review of the literature.

1. CLINICAL OBSERVATION

1.1. Patient presentation

A 58-year-old patient with no previous pathological conditions was referred for prosthetic rehabilitation of the maxillary right molar region.

1.2. Clinical examination

1.2.1. Exo-oral examination

No particularities were noted during the exo buccal examination.

1.2.2. Endo buccal examination

At the endo-buccal examination, hygiene was good, the restoration implanted in the maxillary right molar area was lost and the implants in the regions of the maxillary second premolars and second right molars were affected by severe peri-implantitis.

1.3. Additional examinations

Panoramic radiography and cone-beam computed tomography (CBCT) revealed several problems in the posterior right area of the maxilla:

-   Insufficient bone volume for conventional implant placement due to sinus pneumatisation

-   The restoration in the maxillary right molar region was lost, and the implants in the maxillary second premolar and right molar regions showed severe peri-implantitis.

-   In addition, the implant in the region of the maxillary right first molar failed to osteointegrate and was moved into the maxillary sinus.

^ The two implants in the maxillary second premolar and right second molar regions were surgically removed due to peri-implantitis. Subsequently, a plan was developed to remove the displaced implant in the maxillary sinus using a lateral window approach.

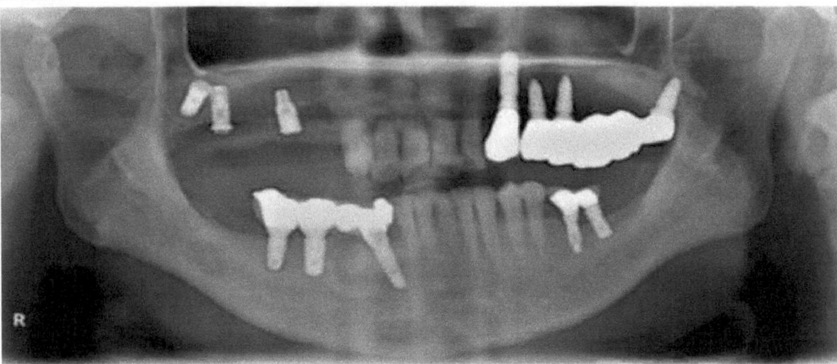

Figure 1: Preoperative panoramic radiograph [55].

1.4. Diagnosis

Lack of sufficient bone height for implant placement between the crete and the sinus floor, with an implant being pushed back into the maxillary sinus.

1.5. Therapeutic decision

Sinus enhancement via the lateral approach after removal of the implant pushes back into the sinus.

1.6. Operating stages

к Anaesthesia

Infiltration of the anterolateral aspect of the maxilla and right palate using an anaesthetic solution

к Incisions

к Detachment

к Osteotomy

An oval-shaped bone window was created and separated from the lateral wall of the maxillary sinus using an 'off-the-wall' osteotomy technique10. The two implants affected by peri-implantitis were removed,

к Sinus membrane detachment

The sinus membrane was lifted and deliberately perforated. The implant in the sinus cavity was removed through the perforation. Finally, the size of the perforation was measured at approximately 1.5 cm in maximum diameter.

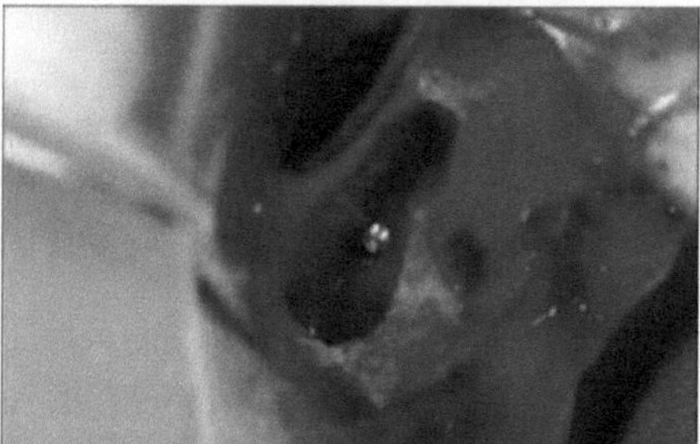

Figure 2: Intraoperative clinical photograph showing repair of a large perforation using rigid intrasinus fixation and stabilisation of a resorbable barrier membrane with a titanium screw [55].

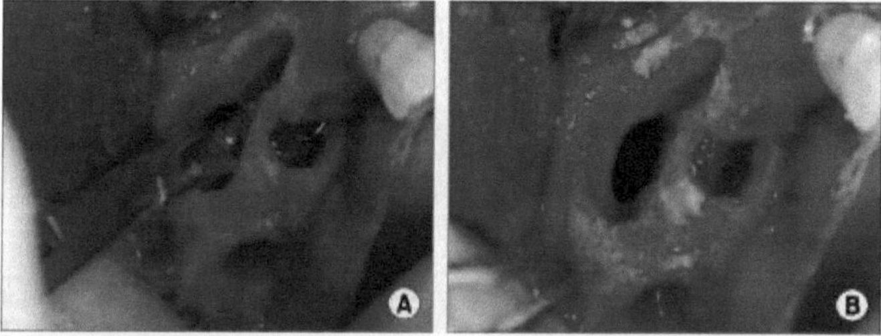

Figure 3: Peroperative clinical photographs. A. The implant, which had been displaced into the sinus cavity, was removed using hemostatic forceps through the perforated sinus membrane. B. A large perforation of the sinus membrane was identified and measured to be approximately 1.5cm in maximum diameter [55].

κ Sinus filling

A semi-rigid, resorbable 3.0cm x 4.0cm collagen barrier membrane (OssMem Hard; Osstem) was asymmetrically designed so that the longer part could be placed and folded into the medial sinus cavity. A titanium screw (Bone Screw; Osstem) was used to fix and stabilise the collagen membrane to the medial or palatal bone surface of the sinus cavity, ensuring coverage of the puncture zone. For bone grafting, a mixture of lyophilised allograft bone (FDBA, SureOss; HansBiomed) and deproteinised bovine bone mineral (DBBM, A-Oss; Osstem) in a 1:1 ratio was hydrated with saline. The hydrated bone graft material was then gently placed under the collagen membrane until the entire sinus cavity was filled and the collagen membrane extended beyond the upper limit of the bone window osteotomy to confirm the complete seal of the graft material.

Dental implants (TS III SOI; Osstem) with a sandy, acid-etched surface coated with a pH buffering agent to introduce hydrophilic properties, promote osteointegration during the early healing period, and accelerate bone formation, have been placed.

Bone graft material was additionally placed, and the separated bone window was repositioned over the bone graft and covered by the outer part of the collagen membrane. Due to the low initial stability of the implants (<10 Ncm), cover screws were attached and the implants were immersed.

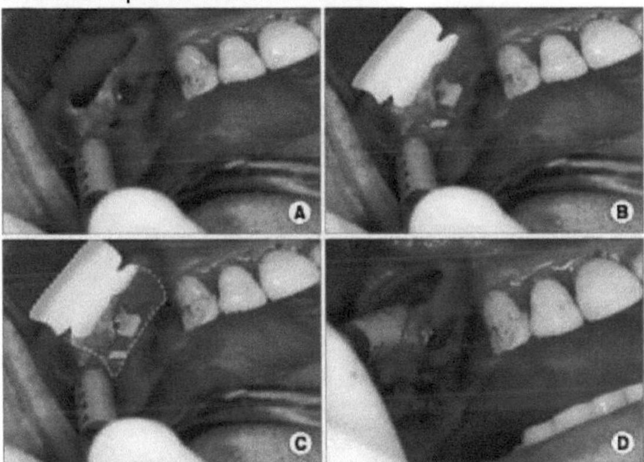

Figure 4: After fixation of the resorbable barrier membrane, bone graft material was inserted into the sinus cavity. A. Bone grafting through the implant drilling site. B, C. Schematic drawings of the design of the resorbable barrier membrane and its rigid intra-sinus fixation with a titanium screw. D. Bone grafting through the lateral window. [55]

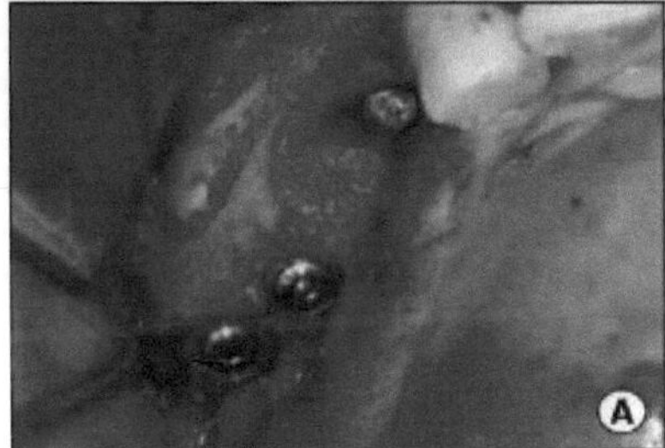

Figure 5: Placement of dental implants after bone grafting. A. A resorbable barrier

κ Sutures

The flap was sutured without tension (Figure 6), and postoperative radiographs were obtained immediately to confirm the proper protection and isolation of the bone graft material by the collagen membrane (Figure 7).

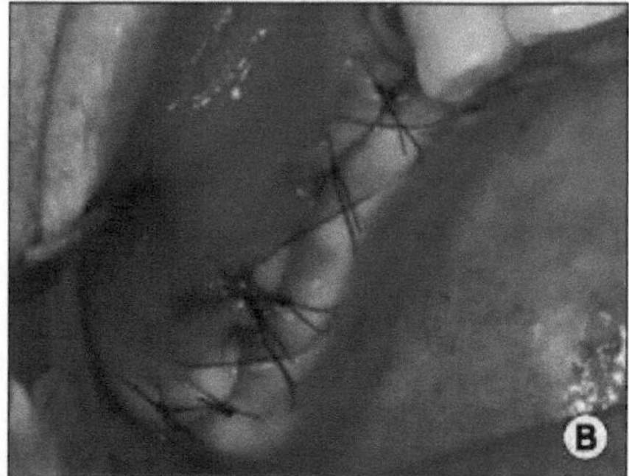

Figure 6: A tension-free suture has been placed [55].

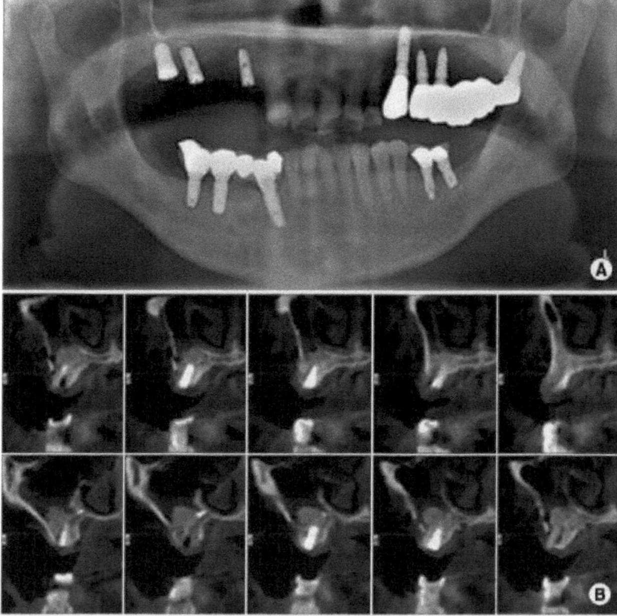

Figure 7: Postoperative radiographs showing that the resorbable barrier membrane, which was internally fixed and stabilised by a titanium screw, maintained its correct position and prevented loss of graft material into the sinus cavity. Panoramic radiograph (A) and cone-beam computed tomography images (B) showing the titanium fixation screw on the medial bone wall of the sinus [55].

к **Prescriptions and post-operations**

The patient received analgesics and antibiotics for 10 days, and a 0.2% chlorhexidine mouthwash was also prescribed three times a day.

The sutures were removed 10 days after surgery. The patient reported no sinus symptoms associated with complications throughout the healing period. After 6 months, the implants were uncovered, and healing abutments were placed. The patient received temporary restorations following the progressive loading protocol.

Finally, 12 months after the initial implant placement and sinus lift procedures, the final restorations were delivered and the patient was satisfied with the result (Fig. 7).

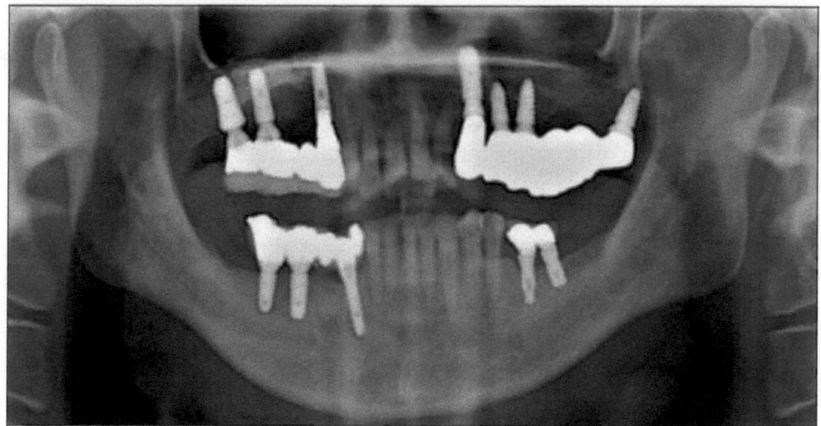

Figure 8: Panoramic radiograph obtained after fitting the final restoration [55].

2. RAISING THE ROOF
OF THE SINUS FLOOR

2.1. Definition of a sinus lift

Sinus lift is a surgical procedure designed to increase the height of the floor of the maxillary sinus. During this procedure, an opening is made in the lateral or alveolar wall of the maxillary sinus to gain access to the interior of the sinus. This opening is then carefully moved and positioned horizontally, creating a doorway to the interior of the sinus (Figure 9) [103].

Once the upper hinge door is correctly positioned, a space is created under the new raised sinus floor. The internal maxillary mucosa, which covers the inside of the sinus, is also lifted to form a cavity of sufficient size. This newly created cavity can be used to place a bone graft or filling material, thereby promoting bone growth and regeneration in the sinus area [103].

It is essential to note that the decision to perform sinus enhancement is based on a thorough evaluation of the clinical situation, including radiographic analysis and discussion with the patient. In this particular case, insufficient residual bone height, measured at less than 5mm, was a decisive factor in opting for sinus lift to improve the outcome and function of dental implants in the posterior maxillary region [103].

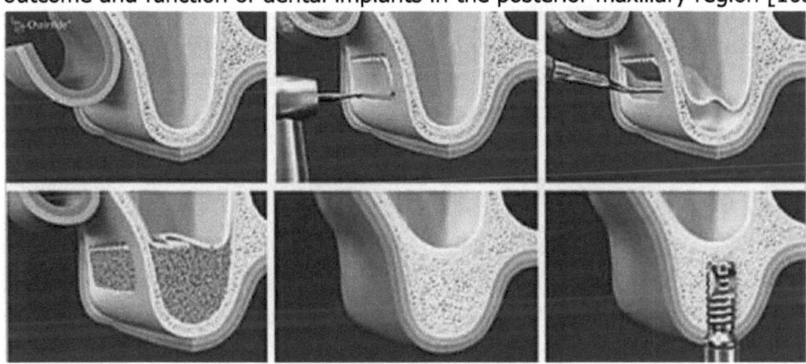

Figure 9: Lateral sinus lift [112].

2.2. History

In 1897, H. Luc [69], a French laryngologist working on the treatment of sinus empyema, proposed a new technique for opening the maxillary sinus by accessing it through the canine fossa. This method involves a 15 mm gingivolabial incision, revealing the outer wall of the sinus. This wall is then perforated at the level of the canine fossa, just above the apices of the premolars. The opening thus created is enlarged, the nasal wall is perforated at its most anterior and most inclined point, and then a trans-sinus meche is inserted [103].

It is important to note that this technique for opening the Highmore antrum was first described by an American in 1893, G.W. Caldwell [16], at the New York Eye Infirmary Congress. Caldwell and Luc worked independently, one in New York and the other in Paris, and the technique for opening the sinus through the canine fossa became known as the Caldwell-Luc technique.

This procedure became the reference method for the treatment of sinus disorders. Later, the development of endoscopic surgery opened up new perspectives and limited the use of the Caldwell-Luc technique [16]. Towards the end of the 60s and during the 70s, a Swedish team in Goteborg developed a system of endosseous implants for total mandibular edentulas. This work led to the publication in 1977 by Branemark and colleagues of an article on the concept of osteointegration of titanium implants, the result of a clinical study with a 10-year follow-up. As a result, these titanium implants were used not only in the mandible, but also in the maxilla, despite the presence of maxillary sinuses and the low sub-sinus height, which limited their indications.

2.2.1.　　Sinus transplants described by Tatum, Boyne and James

In the 1970s, Tatum [98] solved the problem associated with the presence of maxillary sinuses by proposing a surgical technique. After raising a vestibular flap, a bony window is created in the canine fossa while preserving Schneider's membrane. This membrane is carefully detached from the lower part of the sinus, creating an empty space that is filled with autogenous bone chips taken from the iliac crest. The flap is then repositioned and hermetically sutured. This procedure increases the height of the sub-sinus bone, enabling dental implants to be placed in the posterior region of the jaw six months later.

In 1980, Boyne and James [15], followed by Tatum [98] in 1986, were among the first to publish on sinus grafts, and the early 1990s saw a growing interest in this technique. Numerous filling materials appeared.

In 1996, a consensus conference on sinus grafts was held in Massachusetts, reported by Jensen and Schulman [53] in 1998, establishing that sinus grafting is a reliable and proven technique.

However, some have criticised the relatively heavy post-operative sequelae associated with the grafts described by Tatum [72]. In 1994, Summers [96] proposed an alternative approach using osteotomes to lift the sinus floor crestally, a method considered less invasive and associated with milder post-operative effects.

Today, two sinus grafting protocols coexist: the lateral approach initiated by Tatum and the crestal approach with Summers' osteotomes [96]. However, the indications for one or other of these surgical approaches differ.

Maxillary sinus lift can be performed using two main approaches: the lateral approach and the crestal approach. The lateral approach, first described by Tatum in 1976 [98] and published by Boyne and James in 1980, involves the use of autogenous bone as a filling material [15]. Subsequently, in 1994, Summers described another method, called the "osteotome technique", which uses osteotomes of different diameters for a simpler and less invasive approach, allowing simultaneous implant placement [96].

The choice of approach for maxillary sinus lift depends on several factors, including residual bone volume, including residual bone height (RBH) and residual bone septum thickness (BDS), as described in the recent Chiapasco classification. In both techniques, the aim is to achieve guided bone regeneration (GBR). The authors generally use a filling material and a membrane to promote this bone augmentation. A review of the different materials and membranes used in bone regeneration in the posterior region of the maxilla will be discussed in this section in order to gain a better understanding of this problem.

2.3. Indications

Sinus lift is indicated when the residual bone volume is insufficient:

Following the loss of maxillary teeth, physiological changes in the bone and sinuses lead to a reduction in crestal bone height, together with sinus pneumatisation. The classification established by MISCH [72] makes it possible to characterise this bony context by subdividing the residual bone height into four segments (from SA-1 to SA-4), from the top of the bone crest to the sinus floor: (SA = subantral)

- SA-1 is associated with a residual bone height equal to or greater than 12 mm, which allows implants to be fixed without the need for bone augmentation (see Figure 10).

- SA-2 involves a bone height of between 8 and 12 mm, which allows implants to be fixed after prior crestal floor elevation. (See Figure 10)

- SA-3 is associated with a bone height of between 5 and 8 mm, necessitating lateral sinus filling. However, in this situation, the implants can be placed simultaneously with the filling, subject to primary stability. (See Figure 10)

- SA-4 involves a bone height ranging from 0 to 5 mm, also requiring grafting via a lateral approach. In this case, however, a second surgical stage is required to place the implants. (See Figure 10)

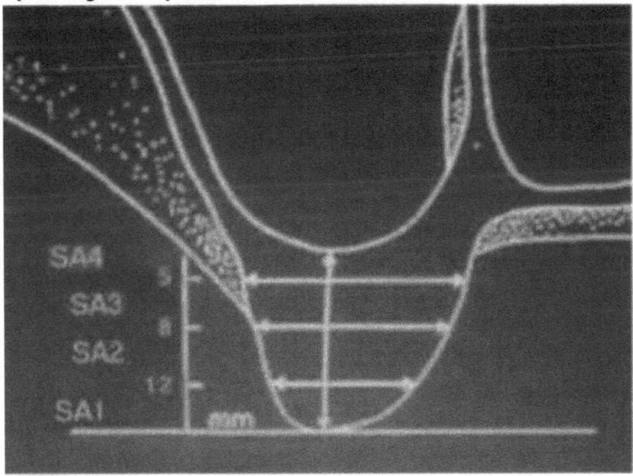

Figure 10: MISH classification according to residual bone height [79].

2.4. Contraindications

2.4.1.   General contraindications

The main contraindications are

- The risk of group A infectious endocarditis [47],
- Previous treatment with intravenous bisphosphonates [2].
- Previous cervico-facial radiotherapy, with a total dose exceeding 60 Gray [5],
- Immunodeficiency, with a CD4 count of less than 400/mm3,
- Bleeding risks of all kinds (hemostasis disorders or anticoagulant/platelet anti-aggregant medication),
- Unbalanced diabetes,
- Bone disease (Paget's disease, fibrodysplasia),
- Allergies or intolerance to anaesthetic products,
- Addictions (alcohol, drugs, tobacco) [57]
- Psychological disorders.

In all cases, close collaboration with the attending physician and the ENT must enable a meticulous assessment of the situation, in order to rule out the potential risks associated with a deterioration in the patient's general condition.

2.4.2.   Local contraindications

The local contraindications commonly taken into account are as follows [57]:
- Acute maxillary sinusitisë
- Cysts or tumours of the maxilla
- Severe or untreated periodontal disease
- Sinus infections of periodontal or endodontic origin (aspergillosis, periodontal cyst)
- Obstruction of the ostio-meatic defiles
- Excessive inter-crest distance.
- Sinus hypoplasia or aplasia
- Oroantral fistula

It is important to ensure that the patient is cooperating properly with regard to oral hygiene and compliance with post-operative recommendations, in order to minimise any complications that may arise.

To investigate these local contraindications, it is essential to have CT scan data covering the entire sinus cavity, enabling a complete and systematic examination of the sinus.

2.5. Sinus lift techniques

There are currently two widely used techniques for maxillary sinus lift.
- The lateral route: a direct conventional method.
- By crestal route: an indirect, less invasive method.

2.5.1.   Pre-surgical assessment

The aim of the pre-surgical assessment is to carry out a complete analysis of all the patient's individual factors in order to define an appropriate treatment plan. It takes into account the patient's anatomical, physiological, emotional and economic imperatives, as well as the practitioner's surgical and prothetic imperatives.

This assessment takes place during a preoperative consultation and follows the following stages [4,81]:
1. Taking into account the patient's requests and expectations.

2. Assessment of patient motivation and cooperation.

3. Assessment of the patient's lifestyle, particularly with regard to smoking habits and other addictions.

4. Study of the medical questionnaire to identify the patient's pathologies, medications, allergies and medical and surgical antecedents.

5. Assessment of individual risk factors and, if necessary, contact with the patient's GP.

6. Detailed extra-oral examination, including observation of facial symmetry, harmony of the facial layers, morphology of the lips and smile.

7. Detailed intra-oral examination, including assessment of oral hygiene, periodontal health, the state of the teeth, edentulous areas, inter-arch relationships, occlusion and the presence of any nausea reflex.

8. Additional radiographic examinations to obtain further information.

9. Photographs and impressions to create study models.

10. Drawing up a treatment plan tailored to the patient's needs and providing an estimate detailing the proposed interventions.

This comprehensive assessment enables the practitioner to make informed decisions and tailor treatment to the specific needs of each patient.

2.5.2. Radiological check-up

A thorough radiological examination is of crucial importance in the planning of any surgical procedure, particularly in the case of sub-sinus filling. Its purpose is to confirm the appropriateness and feasibility of the operation, to provide detailed information on the local anatomical structures (such as bone structure, volume, density, anatomical obstacles, as well as nerve and vascular structures), and to highlight the specific characteristics of the sinuses (volume, partitioning, residual apex, mucosal pathology).

The range of examinations available has grown with the technological and computer revolution and comprises two aspects:

- Two-dimensional images (intra-oral radiography, panoramic, Blondeau, profile teleradiography),

- Three-dimensional imaging (scanner or DM. MRI and more recently CBCT).

The standard radiographic exploration protocol for sinus filling and pre-implant planning is based on the most recent recommendations from researchers and the French National Authority for Health (HAS) [78]. It initially involves panoramic radiography or orthopantomography (OPT), followed by cone-beam computed tomography (CBCT).

к Panoramic cliche

Panoramic radiography or orthopantomography (OPT) should be used as the first line of defence because of its ease of access, low exposure to radiation and wide field of exploration. This examination provides an overall, synthetic view of the oral cavity and the main bone and dental structures [17]. It is the recommended preliminary examination for a new patient's first visit.

However, it should be noted that panoramic radiography does not provide a quantitative or qualitative assessment of the volume of bone available for implantation or intrasinus grafting. The measurements that can be made are limited to bone height. **κ TDM**

Cone-Beam or CBCT is currently emerging as the reference method for anatomical analysis of implant sites and therapeutic planning [46], surpassing CT due to the advantages inherent in its technology. This technique is based on the digital acquisition of data by scanning a cone-shaped beam of X-rays around the patient, which is then computer-processed to reconstruct the explored volume. This approach makes it possible to navigate through the image in all spatial planes and to create sections of 'interest' for surgery. In addition, it can be coupled with implant simulation software to objectively assess the feasibility of the surgical procedure.

Compared with CT scans, CBCT offers improved spatial resolution with smaller voxels, a radiation dose that is around 25 times lower (for an equivalent volume explored), and above all the ability to adjust the size and resolution of the examination according to the procedure envisaged, whether it be a small volume limited to a single tooth or a large volume encompassing the entire skull.

▶ CBCT

From a clinical point of view, the use of Cone Beam Computed Tomography (CBCT) significantly improves the diagnostic evaluation compared with 2D imaging, by providing additional information on the maxillary sinuses and surrounding structures. This diagnostic data is particularly crucial in conjunction with Sinuslift planning, as a thorough radiological analysis is essential not only for sinus procedures, but also for implant placement. Diagnostic features derived from CBCT images that are potentially clinically relevant to the success of a Sinuslift procedure, and which may remain unsuspected with 2D imaging, include:

- **Anatomy of the maxillary sinus and alveolar crete :**

CBCT provides detailed anatomical information regarding sinus morphology and residual alveolar crevice volume. This information is invaluable in determining the optimal approach for accessing the sinus and assessing the quality of the patient's bone for grafting [84,102] (Figure 11).

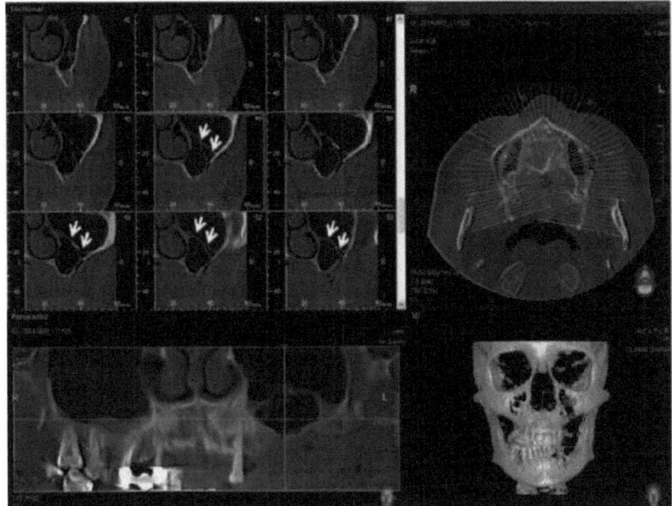

Figure 11: CBCT after sinus lift with bone flap to preserve space (arrows). [59]

- **Relationship of the maxillary sinus to the roots of adjacent teeth :**

The proximity of the dental roots to the schneiderian membrane is assessed to minimise the risk of perforation during sinus lift. The state of health of the adjacent teeth is also examined to detect any pre-existing apical pathologies likely to influence the success of the graft [29,84] .

- **Thickness of the Schneiderian membrane :**

CBCT is a useful tool for measuring the thickness of the sinus membrane [52,56], a factor associated with the risk of perforation [11]. Healthy sinus mucosa has an average thickness of approximately 1 mm, although this may vary considerably from one individual to another [73]. It should be noted that thicknesses greater than 2 mm increase the risk of sinusitis following sinus membrane elevation, and values in excess of 5 mm increase the risk of ostium obstruction [92,99].

- **The maxillary sinus septum [14,89].**

It is frequently observed in approximately one third of patients, a feature ideally identified using three-dimensional (3D) imaging [74]. Understanding the location and morphology of septa is of crucial importance in sinus lift planning, as it is associated with an increased risk of sinus membrane perforation during the procedure. In the presence of a septum, the design of the osteotomy may need to be adapted from a single window technique to two smaller windows on either side of the septum or the use of a W-shaped trap technique. Thus, CBCT imaging plays a key role in developing an appropriate treatment plan [110].

- **The ostium of the maxillary sinus**

It is also of vital importance, as post-sinuslift healing depends to a large extent on adequate drainage into the nasal cavity. Assessing the permeability of the ostium prior to surgery is crucial to avoid complications such as sinusitis or surgical failure. In addition, the search for accessory ostia, which may interfere with sinus ventilation and drainage, is necessary [107].

• **The width of the floor of the maxillary sinus**

The distance and angulation between the lateral and medial walls of the sinus are essential anatomical features to be assessed using CBCT. This makes it possible to determine the potential complexity of the sinus lift procedure, particularly in the case of sinuses that are too narrow or too wide with pronounced angulations. CBCT imaging provides a precise measure of sinus width, guiding the choice of the appropriate surgical approach, for example by avoiding a trap technique that is not recommended for narrow sinuses [18].(Figure 12)

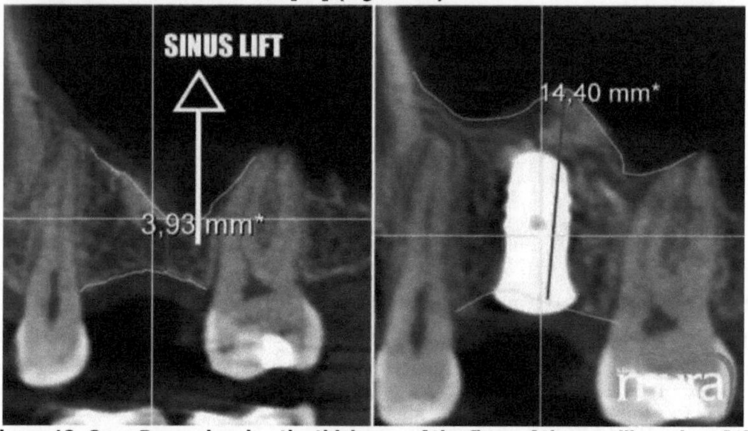

Figure 12: Cone Beam showing the thickness of the floor of the maxillary sinus [4].

• **Thickness of the lateral wall of the maxillary sinus**

This is a crucial parameter to assess at the diagnostic stage with CBCT, because a thick wall complicates the sinus lift, lengthens operating time and increases the risk of perforation. Thus, CBCT imaging is recommended to assist the surgeon in the decision making process, allowing him to assess the thickness of the sinus wall in 3D and to choose the area with the least thickness in order to minimise complications [67].

• **Alveolar-antral artery**

CBCT imaging provides a precise representation of the alveolar-antral artery, allowing optimal surgical planning for sinus access. The alveolar-antral arteries, with a diameter greater than 0.5 mm, are discernible on CBCT, and a diameter greater than 3 mm suggests potentially abundant bleeding. In the presence of this artery at the osteotomy site, the use of a piezoelectric surgical device is recommended. Adjusting the design of the osteotomy window from an oval to a round shape over or either side of this artery may prevent injury [44].

• **Estimating the volume of the graft**

Graft volume estimation, using CBCT images combined with planning software, can be used to measure the volume required for the graft [49]. Precise preoperative planning of graft volume helps to avoid overfilling the sinus, to decide on the ratio between bone and bone substitutes, and to estimate xenograft costs before surgery. In cases of autogenous graft harvesting, prior knowledge of the quantity required is essential to select the optimal donor region, reduce the time and complexity of the procedures, and minimise potential post-operative complications [1].

2.5.3. Protocols

2.5.3.1.   Lateral approach

κ Definition

Described by Hitl TATUM in 1974, this technique uses a variant of the Caldwell-Luc approach to penetrate the sinus. This technique is indicated when the height of the residual crevice is less than 3 mm,

κ Operating protocol for lateral sinus lift [4,65,98].

1.   Local anaesthetic will be administered in the vestibular and palatal region, extending from the canine to the back of the tuberosity. This anaesthetic will be completed by anaesthesia of the crestal and papillary mucosa in the presence of teeth.

2.   An incision trace is made along the crete, with mesial and distal cuts. According to Dr Antoun H [4], it is important to take several factors into account when making the appropriate incision:

-    The size of the maxillary sinus
-    The ideal position for the osteotomy
-    The presence or absence of adjacent teeth
-    Whether or not to place implants intraoperatively
-    The anatomical situation of the maxillary nerve (V2) and its branches, so as not to weigh them down during incision 2.

An incision will be made on the edentulous crete, slightly offset towards the palate, or an intrasulcular incision if teeth are present. This incision should be full-thickness and larger than the planned bone fenestration, extending one centimetre mesially and one centimetre distally.

A mesial relief incision, also full-thickness, will begin at the mesial end of the crestal incision, moving up into the vestibule, cutting through the keratinised gingiva and free mucosa, at a distance from the most anterior area of the future bone window.

A distal offloading incision (which is optional) will be made with care to preserve the vascularisation of the flap.

3.   The full thickness flap is delicately detached to expose the anterolateral wall of the maxilla down to the base of the zygomatic bone. This detachment is carried out while respecting the V2.

4.   A window of bone will be created by osteotomy, which may be oval or rectangular in shape. It will be small enough to ensure the stability of the graft while guaranteeing good vascularisation and healing.

The osteotomy can then be performed in 2 ways:

-    Non-conservative approach to the bone window
-    Conservative approach to the bone window
-    The choice of practitioner depends on the difficulty of the operation (Table 1).

Table 1: Possible types of osteotomy and materials used.

Non-conservative	Curator
Figure 13: Osteotomy using a diamond ball burr [59].	**Figure 14: Osteotomy using a saw-shaped piezoelectric insert [12].**
In this approach, a <u>slice </u>is created to access the sinus. The sinus window can be either detached or reclined inside the sinus.	In this approach, a <u>mini-trench </u>is created. The window is detached, preserved in physiological serum for the duration of the operation and then repositioned at the end of the procedure. The advantage of this technique is that it is more biological and conservative.
Equipment used	
<u>Tungsten ball end mill </u>followed by a <u>diamond end mill </u>mounted on a handpiece	Piezoelectric insert: thin saw-shaped insert (more or less angled)
Ultrasonic (US) diamond ball insert (if the cortex is thin, i.e. <2mm)	
<u>Tungsten ball end mill </u>followed by a <u>US diamond ball insert</u>	

5.   Schneider's membrane will be detached to free the bone window in its lower and proximal parts. Practitioners use a variety of methods to detach the sinus membrane, ranging from piezo surgery to the manual curette. Further debonding involves the use of manual curettes with different angulations. During this procedure, several conditions must be observed to minimise the risk of sinus membrane perforation (Figure 15):

-   The curettes must maintain continuous contact with the bone walls.

-   The convex part of the curette must always be directed towards the sinus mucosa.

-   The detachment must be carried out gradually, gradually loosening the mucosa.

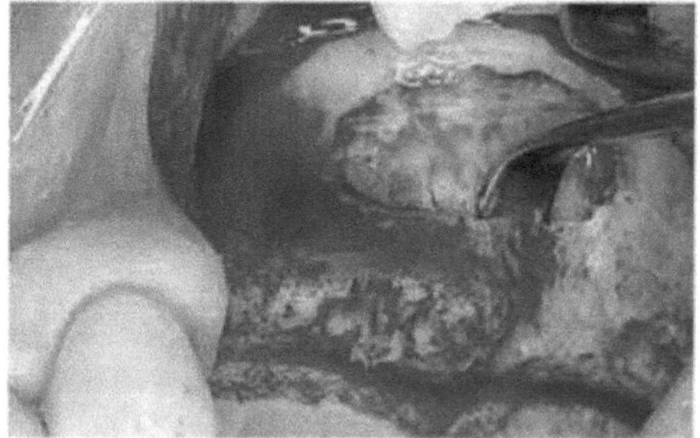

Figure 15: Detachment of the sinus membrane using a curette [31].

6.   The bone window is then lifted upwards, taking the sinus membrane with it, to create a concave bed for the graft, taking care not to obstruct the sinus drainage hole. The membrane must be detached from the medial wall of the sinus to avoid

the formation of a sinus pocket or cul-de-sac.

7.   The graft is carefully prepared by hydrating it with physiological serum or the patient's own blood.

8.   The bone graft will be placed in close contact with the bony walls of the sinus, compact to avoid air pockets or gaps. (Figure 16).

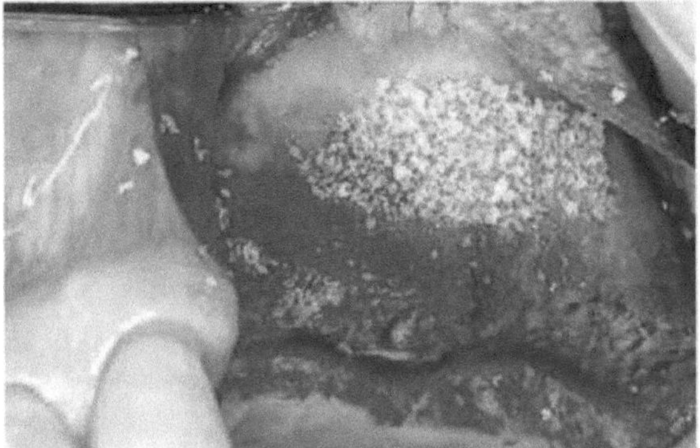

Figure 16: Graft placement [31].

9.   A resorbable collagen membrane, whose surface area exceeds that of the bone window, may be positioned to cover the edges over a distance of 3 mm. The role of this membrane is to stabilise the graft and protect the site (Figure 17).

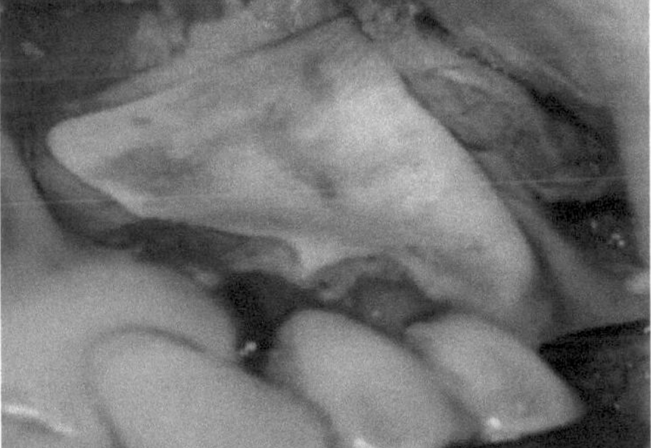

Figure 17: Covering the graft with a resorbable collagen membrane [43].

10. Finally, the flap is repositioned and sutured, ensuring hermetic closure without tension, using discontinuous stitches 5 mm apart with non-absorbable thread (Figure 18).

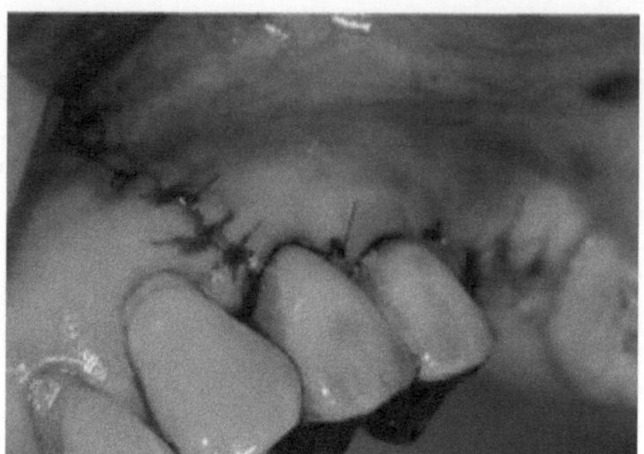
Figure 18: flap replacement and suture [43].

2.5.3.2.   Crestal approach

κ Definition

The crestal approach technique for sinus lift was introduced by Summers [96] in 1994.

Unlike the lateral approach, the crestal approach, also known as Summers surgery, avoids the need for a lateral approach. The sinus is accessed directly from the top of the crete. Using osteotomes of increasing size with blunt tips [96], the sinus membrane is detached vertically, while keeping the membrane raised to encourage the formation of a blood clot. This clot will support colonisation by bone-forming cells, stimulating bone formation.

Although this technique is less invasive than the lateral approach and generally leads to fewer post-operative complications, it does present some challenges. Visibility of the membrane during surgery is limited, which increases the risk of perforation. In addition, the crestal approach is not suitable for all situations, and is mainly indicated when there is a minimum residual bone volume of at least 5 mm [43].

κ The surgical protocol includes the following steps

1) Anaesthesia

2) Preparation of the operating field

3) A crestal incision is made, accompanied by sulcal and/or vertical incisions to expose the bone site. The vestibular and palatal flaps are removed.

4) Initiation of an osteotomy of the crestal bone at the implant site using a ball burr. Osteotomes of increasing diameter are then introduced into the site using a mallet, in successive strokes, to prepare the implant site, raise the sinus floor and create the space required for insertion of the implant (Figure 19). Osteotomes can be angled or straight, and of different diameters (Figure 20) [6,43,96].

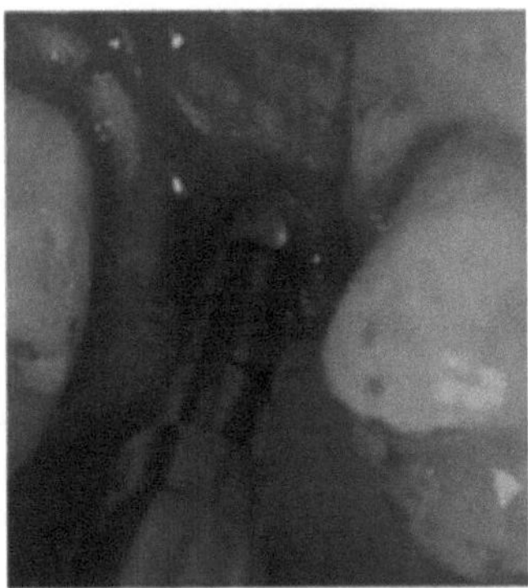

Figure 19: Use of an osteotome to lift the sinus floor [87].

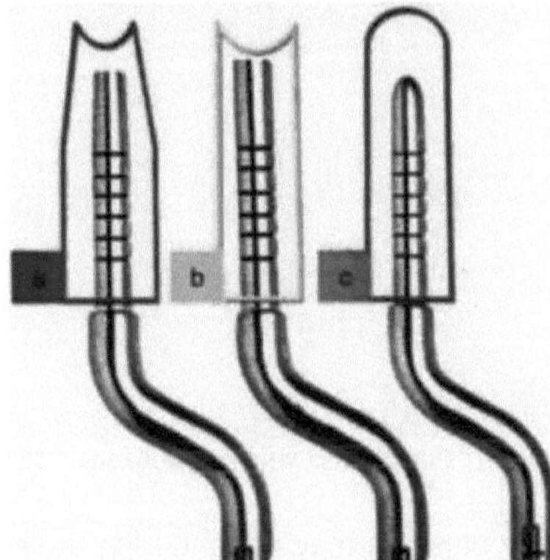

Figure 20: Different osteotomes [118] a) Cylindro-conical osteotome with concave end; b) Cylindrical osteotome with concave end; c) Cylindrical osteotome with rounded convex end.

The depth of the osteotomes is chosen according to the height of the alveolar ridge measured beforehand. The last osteotome should be 1 mm smaller than the implant diameter, while remaining 1 mm from the sinus floor, thus promoting the implant's primary stability. In some difficult cases, an adapted implant drill can be used, stopping 1 mm from the sinus floor, followed by the use of a smaller diameter osteotome [43,98].

5) Check the integrity of the membrane using a depth gauge at the non-traumatic foam end. Resistance should be perceptible to avoid perforating the membrane [96].

6) Instant or delayed implant placement. Insertion can be carried out using a motor to the apical limit of the residual bone void. In order to gently lift the membrane without damaging it, insertion is preferably completed with a torque wrench [6,96].

7) Sutures are made with the operator's choice of composition and size of thread.

Inflammatory sinus polyps, which we discuss here, are outgrowths of the sinus mucosa caused by allergies and infections of the sinus system. These polyps, which are generally benign, may be single or multiple, sometimes measuring up to 5 cm. An isolated sinus polyp is often asymptomatic and is most frequently located on the

21

posterior (92.3%) or lateral (61.5%) wall, more rarely on the sinus floor (38.5%).

2.5.4.   Complications

Complications related to sinus lift surgery can occur at two different times: during surgery (per-operatively) or after surgery (post-operatively). Although these complications are generally rare, it is essential for the practitioner to be aware of them in order to prevent them [4].

Intraoperative complications may include :

-     Perforation of the sinus membrane: This can occur when an attempt is made to lift the membrane, resulting in direct communication between the sinus and the oral cavity. However, this complication can often be managed during the same surgery. (Figure 21)

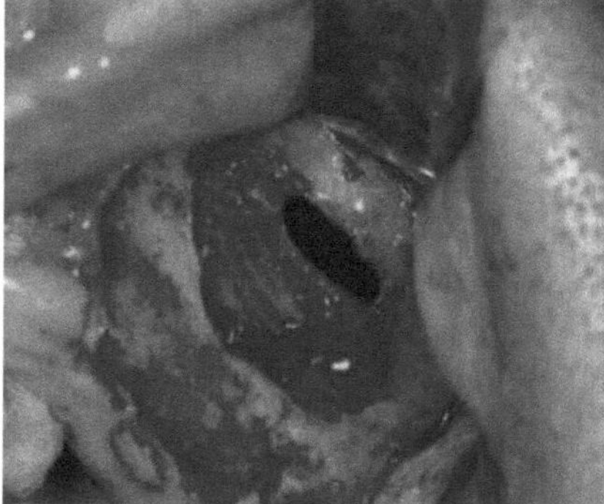

Figure 21: Perforated sinus membrane [85].

-     Haemorrhage: Excessive bleeding may occur during the operation. Good control of hemostasis is necessary to avoid this complication.

-     Lesions of the antral alveolar artery

Post-operative complications may include

-     Subcutaneous haematoma: An accumulation of blood under the skin may occur after surgery, causing swelling and pain.

-     Hemosinus: This is bleeding into the sinuses, which can lead to symptoms such as epistaxis (nosebleed).

-     Bucco-sinusal communication: A persistent opening between the sinus and the oral cavity can lead to air and fluid leakage, disrupting healing and increasing the risk of infection.

-     Displacement of the grafted bone substitute: The filling material used may move from its intended position, affecting the success of the graft.

-     Suture rupture with exposure of the surgical site: If the sutures do not hold in place, the surgical site may be exposed, increasing the risk of infection.

-     Graft infection: Any surgical procedure carries a risk of infection, and sinus lift surgery is no exception.

-     Acute or chronic sinusitis : Lifting the sinus can cause inflammation of the sinus mucosa, leading to acute or chronic sinusitis.

It is essential that the practitioner takes all the necessary measures to minimise the risk of complications and follows the appropriate post-operative protocols to ensure a successful and healing operation.

2.5.5. Risk factors for perforation

2.5.5.1. Sinus polyp [24,91].

It is important to note that the presence of inflammatory sinus polyps is not necessarily a contraindication to sinus filling, provided that they do not block the middle meat. However, sinusoscopy is recommended to assess the potential risk, as the presence of polyps can make membrane detachment more complex and increase the risk of secondary ostium blockage.

If the middle meat is blocked by a polyp, surgery will be necessary before considering a sinus graft.

2.5.5.2. Intrasinus septum [41,42,54,66,74,80,86,104,106].

Intrasinusal septa, also known as Underwood's septa, form bony walls that partially or totally divide the sinus cavities, creating small accessory sinuses (see Figure 22). These septa act as bone reinforcements during the dental phase of mastication and appear to diminish progressively with tooth loss.

Some authors have developed a classification of septa according to their origin:

- The primary septa form parallel to the development of the maxilla and are present during the dental phase.

- Secondary septa appear following tooth loss, as a result of selective resorption of the sinus floor, and take the form of protrusions and depressions.

The primary septa are significantly longer than the secondary septa, and are capable of causing complete division of the sinus.

These primary septa can take a variety of forms, depending on their size and orientation (sagittal or frontal), and they can constitute an obstacle to the preservation of Schneider's membrane.

According to studies, these septa are present in around 28% of cases (24% to 32% depending on the study) and are visible on cone-beam computed tomography (CBCT). It is essential to use CBCT to diagnose intrasinusal septa, as studies have shown false negatives with panoramic dentomaxillary radiographs (21% false negatives compared with CBCT and 2D radiographs).

The preferred location of the septa is on the maxillary first molars (28.6%), maxillary second molars (22.9%) and maxillary second premolars (22.9%). Their average height varies from 2.8 to 8.1 mm.

It is important to note that there is no correlation between the presence of septa and factors such as gender, age or coastline, although there is a slightly higher prevalence in the Asian population (22.9%). Septa are generally individual rather than multiple within the same sinus (two septa in 3.7% of cases, three or more septa in 0.5% of cases), with a more frequent transverse than sagittal orientation. In addition, their thickness tends to increase from the lateral to the medial portion.

These septa may be unilateral in around 65% of cases, but also bilateral in around 35%. Their presence can complicate sinus elevation using a lateral approach, increasing the risk of Schneider's membrane perforation.

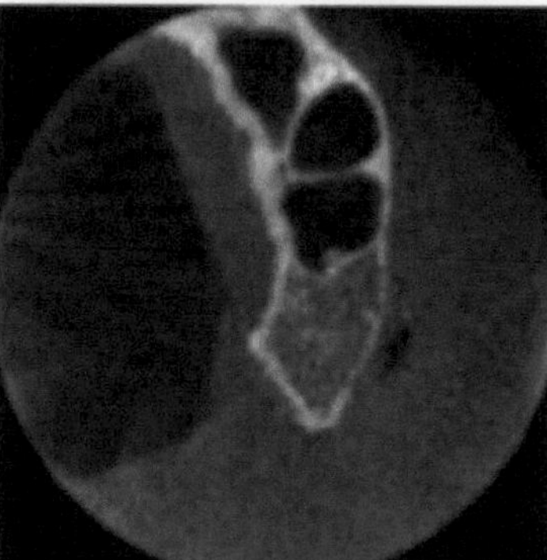

Figure 22. Neck view of intrasinus septa [106].

κ Partial perpendicular septa [80,106].

Partial perpendicular septa divide the sinus cavities only partially. They may be transverse (latero-medial) in 87.6% of cases or sagittal (antero-posterior) in 11.1% of cases.

Partial perdicular septa with a transverse orientation, located anteriorly to the zygomatic process and measuring less than 6 mm in height, can be integrated into the sinus filling by creating a single lateral access window. However, when the height is greater than 6 mm, two windows are required on either side of the septum.

In a position posterior to the zygomatic process, management of these septa is a moderate difficulty, depending also on their height. If the bone is less than 6mm high, a single lateral access window is generally adequate. However, when the height is greater than 6 mm, this single window is completed by removing the septum using a diamond insert.

Partial perpendicular septa oriented sagittally are considered a major difficulty for sinus filling. For an anterior-posterior septum less than 6 mm high, a traditional lateral access window is used. However, if the septum is higher than 6 mm, a crestal access window is required to detach the um and lift the sinus membrane.

In conclusion, the presence of multiple septa also represents a significant challenge, requiring the creation of several access windows. However, it is essential to stress that multiple septa within a single sinus are very rare, representing around 4.2% of cases (Table II).

Table II. Classification of the different septa and suggested management [106].

Classification	Location	Number	Orientation	Size (mm)	Proposed therapeutic approach
Simple					
a	Antero-zygomatic	1	Mediolaterale	<6	1 access window
b	Antero-	1	Mediolaterale	>6	2 windows

24

	zygomatic				
Moderee					
a	Postero-zygomatic	1	Mediolaterale	<6	1 access window or crestal approach
1 window					
b	Postero-septum	1	Mediolaterale	>6	access and zygomatica removal of the
Difficult					
a	Antero-zygomatic or postero-zygomatic	1	Antero-posterior	<6	1 access window
b	Antero-zygomatic or postero-zygomatic	1	Antero-posterior	>6	1 crestal access window
c	Antero-zygomatic or postero-zygomatic	>2	Mediolaterale		Multiple windows

κ Partial horizontal septa (2700,2800)

Partial horizontal septa are uncommon, occurring in around 1.3% of cases. They are characterised by a horizontal extension from the palatine bone and the inferior horn, always running horizontally towards the skull.

These septa generally have no impact on sinus filling if they are above the level of the graft. However, if they are horizontal and below the level of the graft, they can impede sinus drainage, potentially leading to graft failure.

κ Complete septa [32,80]

Complete septa are uncommon, accounting for only 0.3% of cases. They are distinguished by their ability to divide the sinus cavity into two distinct parts: a large anterior sinus and a small posterior (accessory) sinus (Figure 23).

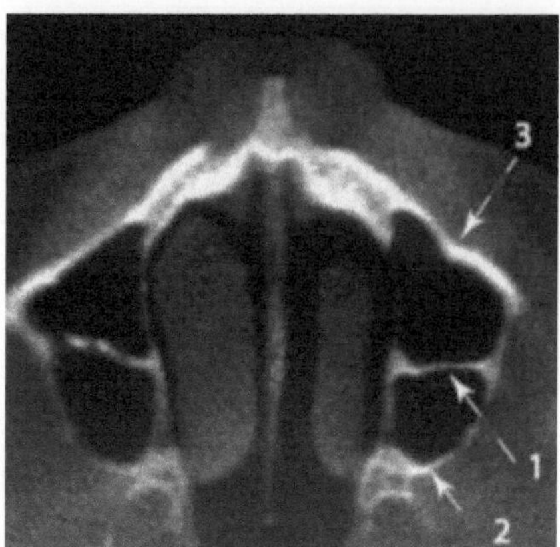

**Figure 23. CBCT cross-sectional image showing: 1 = complete septum ;
2 = lateral wall ; 3 = posterior wall [32]**

2.5.5.3. Angulation between vestibular and palatal walls (width of sinus floor) [7,21,58,90,105].

The angle created by the vestibular and palatal walls of the maxillary sinus is a significant risk factor for perforation. This angle influences the medio-lateral width of the sinus floor. The more acute the angle, the narrower the sinus, which increases the risk of perforation of the sinus membrane (see Table III).

A sinus classification based on this angulation has been proposed by the team of Drs. Wiley and John :

- Below 30° (around 4.8% of the population)
- Between 31° and 60° (around 42.8% of the population)
- Above 61° (around 52.4% of the population)

**Table III. Impact of sinus floor angulation on sinus
membrane perforations in sinus fillers [90].**

Angulation between walls		
<30° 30°< x < 60° >60° vestibular and palatal (°)		
Percentage of perforations 37.5%28 .	5%0	

It is important to note that no relationship was established between this angle, the age of the patients or their sex.

2.5.5.4. Low membrane thickness [8].

The thickness of the sinus membrane varies both between and within individuals, depending on the different anatomical areas. It is also relevant to note that this membrane tends to be generally thicker in men than in women.

As this is visible on three-dimensional X-ray examination (CBCT), it is recommended that this is carried out prior to surgery to allow a thorough pre-surgical analysis.

The incidence of sinus membrane perforation varies according to the surgical approach adopted. For example, with a lateral approach, the risk of sinus membrane perforation is estimated at between 20 and 44%, whereas with a crestal approach, the risk varies between 0 and 25%.

These variations are linked to differences in thickness between the different approach zones.

A thin sinus membrane (less than 1 mm) will naturally have less resistance to perforation. However, it is important to stress that even a pathologically thick sinus membrane (greater than 2 mm) will have less resistance to perforation due to alteration of its internal structure.

(pseudostratified ciliated epithelium, less resistant connective tissue and lamina propria). Consequently, for membranes of atypical thickness, the risk of perforation is multiplied, up to two to three times that observed for membranes of normal thickness. (Table IV)

Table IV. Classification of sinus membrane thicknesses and percentage of perforations (after: WEN et al., 2014).

Group	Membrane thickness	Average	Maximum (mm)	Minimum (mm)	Percentage	Proportion of perforations (%)
A	<1mm	0,64 +/0,19	0,9	0,2	38,92	18,06
B	1 a <2mm	1,36+/ 0,27	1,9	1,0	35,14	13,85
C	>2mm	4,07 +/ 2,88	11,8	2,0	25,95	20,83

2.5.5.5. Former CBS [11]

An oral-sinus communication can occur during oral surgery procedures, such as tooth extractions. In these situations, the sinus membrane is able to heal later, leaving only a scar at the site of the perforation.

However, this scarred area represents a zone of reduced resistance within the sinus membrane, making it a high-risk zone in the event of sinus elevation with membrane detachment. It is therefore essential to take this information into account during the medical examination prior to any operation.

3. INTRA-OPERATIVE MANAGEMENT PERFORATION

The classification of sinus membrane perforations, developed by Fugazzotto and Vlassis [37] in 1999 and again in 2003, is based on a clinical study of several cases of perforation. The aim of this classification is to categorise perforations into different classes according to their specific location in the sinus membrane, and to assess the associated repair options [37].

Regardless of the classification or extent of the breach in the sinus membrane, certain steps must be taken before any attempt is made to repair it. Once a tear has been discovered, it is crucial not to manipulate the sinus membrane any further, so that the size and location of the break can be accurately assessed.

It is recommended to improve the mucoperiosteal flap, if necessary, by extending the incisions and detachment in order to optimise access to the surgical site and improve intra-sinus visibility. Once these measures have been taken, the perforation can be assessed, classified and finally repaired.

κ Class I

Perforations located in the upper 1/3 of the access window; not necessarily requiring further treatment as the debonding continues (figure 24).

Once the perforation has been identified, the surgeon must proceed with the repair, taking care to avoid excessive pressure during detachment in the lesioned area. High pressure could aggravate the tear. Debonding continues in the conventional way, keeping the instrument in contact with the underlying bone. This disbonding causes the membrane to push back apically, forming folds that spontaneously seal the tear, providing a Class I perforation "seal". A collagen or PRP membrane can then be placed over the lesioned area. If immediate implantation was planned pre-operatively, it can be carried out during the same session.

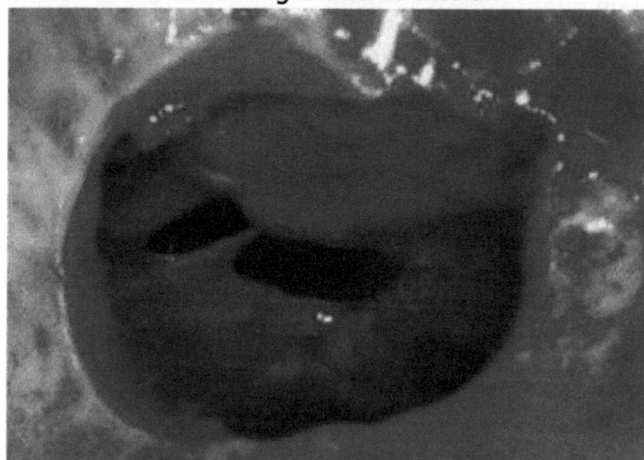

Figure 24: Class I perforation [12].

κ Class II

Perforations located in the lower 2/3 of the access window, either mesial or distal. This class can be divided into two subclasses II.A and II.B, depending on the presence of residual alveolar bone in the vicinity. In this class, the aim is twofold: to repair the defect while continuing the operation.

κ Class II.A

These perforations are located at a distance of 5 mm or more from the walls of the sinus proper (Figure 25). Repair of the perforation is possible in these cases if the sinus is wide or if the bone window is small.

For class II.A perforations, located at a distance of 5 mm or more from the sinus walls, repair begins by increasing the vestibular osteotomy to expose a healthy sinus membrane. Detachment continues cautiously, and apical displacement of the membrane forms folds to reduce the size of the breche.

If a small lesion of less than 2-3 mm persists, a collagen membrane can be used. If the lesion is larger than 3 mm, a porcine membrane (Bioguide, Luitpold, Inc., Shirley, NY) or a bioresorbable membrane (Resolut adapt, W.L. Gore and associates, Inc., Flagstaff, AZ) is used. This membrane is trimmed to be larger than the perforated area, resting on a healthy membrane. In these cases, the immediate implantation planned preoperatively is still possible.

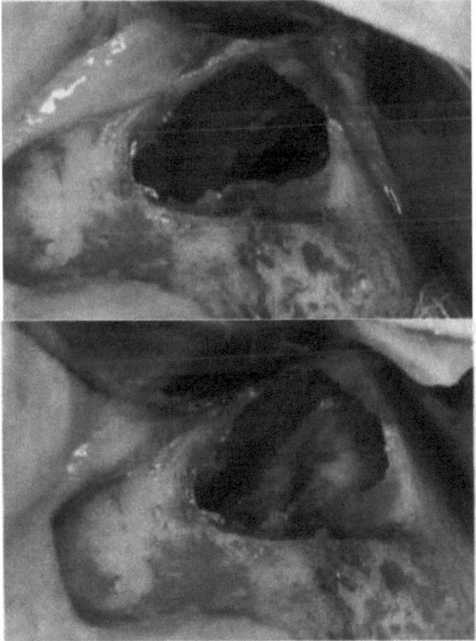

Figure 25: Perforation of the class II sinus membrane and repair with a membrane [12].

κ Class II.B

In the case of perforations less than 4 mm from the sinus wall, increasing the osteotomy is not possible without the risk of increasing the size of the lesion. In these cases, the aim of the repair is to create a "new membrane" to provide a new container for the biomaterial.

A bioresorbable membrane (BioOss, Osteohealth Co., Shirley, NY) is trimmed and then folded back on itself. It is delicately inserted into the sinus cavity previously created, with the edges of the membrane resting on the surrounding alveolar bone outside the sinus. It is then fixed to the alveolar walls using fixation screws (Freos Tacks, Nobel Biocare, Loma Linda, CA). A curette is used to mould the membrane to the shape of the intrasinus cavity, creating sufficient space to receive and contain the biomaterial.

Following this procedure, only the filling is carried out, followed by a healing period of 6 to 8 months. At this point, the implants can be inserted.

κ Class III

These are perforations that are located in the centre of the osteotomy window, and the repair is similar to that of Class II.B. In these cases, the perforation may have existed prior to the operation (following traumatic tooth extraction, bucco-sinusal communication, pneumatisation of the sinus, etc.) or may be the result of a poorly performed osteotomy. In some cases, maxillary resorption may be so extensive that the buccal mucosa is in direct contact with the sinus membrane. The repair procedure involves the use of a bioresorbable membrane that is cut and folded on itself, and inserted delicately into the sinus cavity. The membrane is fixed to the alveolar walls with fixation screws, creating a space for the biomaterial. After filling, there is a healing period of 6 to 8 months before the implants are placed.

The purpose of the repair procedure is to close the perforation in the membrane to prevent the biomaterial from dispersing into the sinus, which could lead to obstruction of the ostium and/or cause sinusitis.

As a result, the following treatment approaches have been observed to achieve adequate implant survival rates:

-    Perforations of less than 5 mm can be treated by folding the membrane itself [10,77] or with resorbable sutures [48,77].

-    When perforations are between 5 and 10 mm, the most widely recommended treatment is the use of a slow resorbing collagen membrane [10,35,36,48,75], which allows regeneration while facilitating closure of the defect. Adjuvant treatment may include the use of a resorbable hemostatic agent [75] or resorbable sutures [10,35] or PRF [76]. PRF activates the vascular system and promotes angiogenesis. As FRP is highly resistant due to its fibrin network, it can prevent graft particles from escaping into the sinus [76]. In perforations of up to 10 mm, it is considered possible to continue with the MSFA procedure and even place the implants simultaneously [48].

-    When perforations of more than 10 mm occur, a combination of laminar bone and a slowly resorbing collagen membrane should be used [48]. In this case, it is advisable to place implants at a later stage [36]. These treatment approaches are based on the size of the membrane perforation and aim to ensure adequate implant survival in different clinical situations.

3.1. Repair techniques

3.1.1.   Therapeutic abstention

3.1.1.1.   Indication [37,48,71]

If the sinus membrane is perforated during submaxillary grafting, the therapeutic approach may vary depending on the size and location of the perforation. According to the 2003 classification by Fugazzato and Vlassis [37], when the perforation is less than 5 mm in diameter and extends towards the upper edge of the osteotomy (class 1 in Fugazzato's classification), a therapeutic option may be to abstain. In this situation, a simple membrane detachment can be performed to promote sealing at the edges, resulting from the folding of the membrane on itself.

Nasal endoscopy can reveal membrane healing after around 6 weeks, especially in the case of small perforations, as demonstrated by the work of Dr Baumann's team in 1999. This conservative approach allows natural recovery of the membrane, promoting healing without aggressive surgery.

3.1.1.2.   Abstention without postponement of bone grafting [19]

In the case of a perforation of the lower sinus membrane of less than 2 mm, one therapeutic option is to abstain without postponing bone grafting. In this situation, it is recommended that the membrane be detached on either side of the perforation. This procedure allows the membrane to fold in on itself, helping to close the perforation. The graft material is then delicately inserted and compressed to fill the newly created subcutaneous space. The aim of this approach is to encourage natural healing while maintaining the continuity of the bone grafting process (Figure 26).

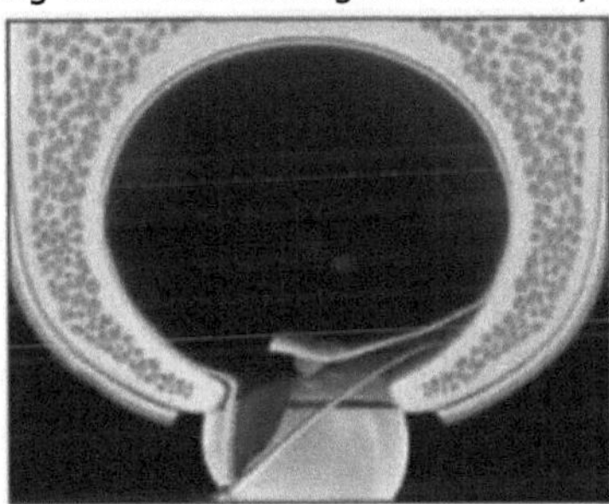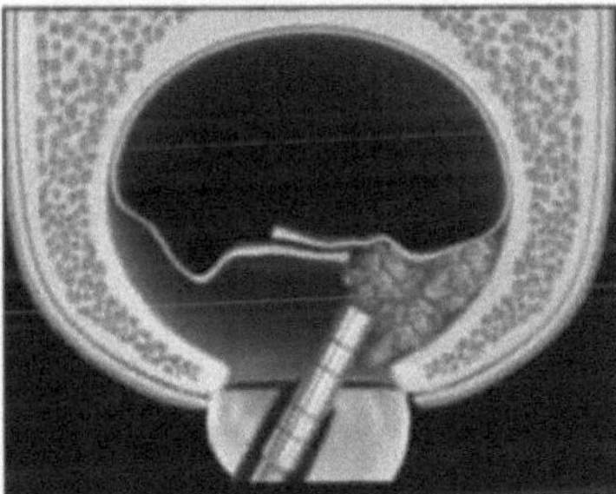

Figure 26 : Detachment of the perforated sinus membrane and concomitant bone graft [19].

3.1.1.3.   Abstention with postponement of bone grafting [13]

Some authors, including Antoun [4], recommend postponing bone grafting if a perforation is detected during site preparation. This postponement is generally fixed at a few months, often between 3 and 4 months. This decision stems from the potential intraoperative treatment difficulties associated with the perforation, as well as the relative imprecision in the immediate management of the situation. By delaying the graft, practitioners aim to create more favourable conditions for the success of the operation, while allowing the perforated area to stabilise and heal before the bone graft is undertaken.

3.1.2.   Mucosal sutures

3.1.2.1.   Indication [48]

When the membrane is torn, and if the perforation is less than 5mm in diameter, suturing with resorbable suture may be considered (resorbable sutures are generally preferred to avoid the need for a second operation to remove the sutures).

It is important to note the difficulty associated with this technique, mainly due to the lack of access and the thinness of the membrane, making it easily tearable. This carries a potential risk of increasing the initial diameter of the perforation, adding to the complexity of managing this delicate surgical situation.

3.1.2.2.   Operating technique [23,48,70,85].

If the perforation of the membrane occurs close to the upper edge of the lateral access window, the membrane may be sutured to the bone wall using a Vycril 6/0 resorbable suture. It is important to continue detaching the membrane beforehand in order to limit the tension exerted on it during suturing.

The cortex is then drilled at the upper edge of the lateral access window using a carbide burr. This is followed by O-shaped sutures with 6/0 Vycril resorbable suture, using an atraumatic round needle and a Castroviejo-type surgical needle holder. The first stitch is positioned approximately 4-5 mm from the caudal edge of the membranous perforation, allowing initial craniocaudal approximation of the perforation edges without tension. Next, mesio-distal stitches are placed every 4-5 mm cranially. The last stitch is passed through the perforation previously made close to the access window, thus securing the sinus membrane to the jawbone. It should be noted that, depending on the orientation of the perforation, this technique can be adapted, for example by making several transcortical perforations to create several suspended points in the case of a mesio-distal oriented perforation. (figure 28, 27)

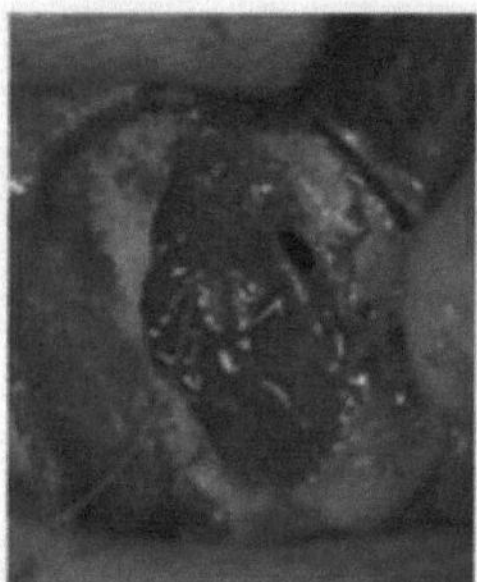 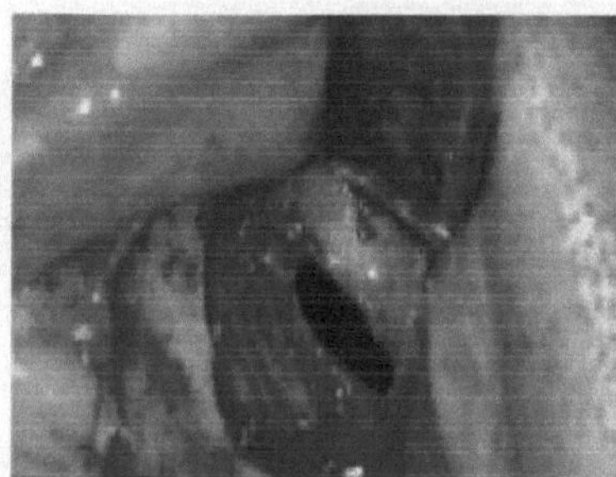

Figure 27: Suture of the perforation [70] Figure 28: Perforation of the membrane [70].

3.1.3.   Fibrin-rich plasma

3.1.3.1.   Indications for the use of FRP in membrane repair [8,13].

Platelet-rich fibrin (PRF) membranes can be used to occlude sinus membrane perforations in pre-implant surgery, particularly for small perforations less than 5mm in diameter. Their biological properties, ease of handling and application, and moderate cost make them a preferred method for repairing membrane perforations (see Figure 29).

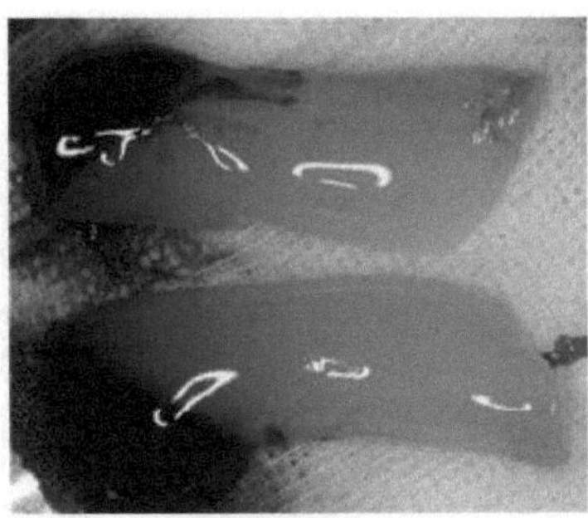

Figure 29: FRP [113]

The use of a FRP membrane requires prior preparation, including drawing blood from the patient and centrifuging the tube to obtain the membrane. Once the perforation has been identified, the membrane is further peeled off around the perforation to reduce stress on the membrane and make it easier to fold. The FRP membrane obtained by centrifugation is then applied to the perforation.

The biological properties of the FRP membrane make it naturally adherent to the sinus membrane, helping to obstruct the perforation and accelerate the healing process. The sinus can then be filled using conventional methods.

The biological characteristics of the FRP membrane make it naturally adherent to the sinus membrane, promoting effective obliteration of the perforation and accelerating the healing process. Once the perforation has been treated, the sinus filling procedure can then be carried out in the conventional way.

3.1.4. Resorbable collagen membrane

3.1.4.1. Composition

Collagen membranes, such as BioGide®, used to repair sinus membrane perforations, are always resorbable. This eliminates the need for subsequent surgery to remove the membrane. The collagen they contain can come from two sources:

- Porcine, bovine or equine origin (peritoneum, pericardium, dermis). Collagen of porcine origin is widely used because of its similarity to human collagen.

- Human origin (placenta, dura mater).

3.1.4.2. Properties [88]

The collagen present in these membranes offers the advantage of being chemotactic for the regenerative cells, thus stimulating the healing of the sinus membrane that was previously perforated. What's more, the collagen membrane is biocompatible, meaning that it is well tolerated by the body and poses no risk of rejection for the patient.

3.1.4.3. Indications [48,82]

In the context of sinus membrane perforations during pre-implant surgery, as in the method used in the reported clinical case, repair can be carried out using resorbable collagen membranes. Several scenarios can be envisaged:

- Perforation of the sinus membrane less than 5 mm in diameter: the perforation is covered with a collagen membrane.

- Perforation of the sinus membrane between 5 and 10 mm: the perforation can be covered with a collagen membrane, with the bone lamella of the lateral access window applied against this membrane.

3.1.4.4. Operating technique [45,82]

The process of repairing a sinus membrane perforation begins by detaching the membrane around the perforation to minimise stress on it. A collagen membrane is then cut to a size much larger than that of the perforation, and inserted into the sub-sinus space thus created. It is applied against the sinus membrane at the level of the perforation. The substitute biomaterial is then delicately introduced, with or without immediate implantation. Finally, the flap is sutured in the conventional manner (Figure 30).

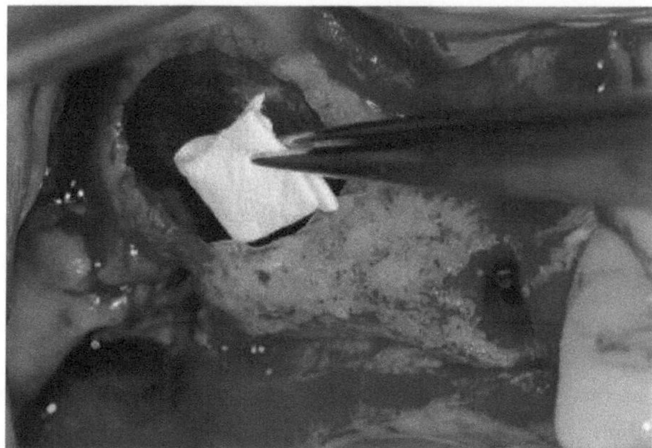

Figure 30: Placement of a resorbable collagen membrane [115].

3.1.5. Rotation of the bone lamella from the lateral access window

3.1.5.1. Indications [48]

In the case of a sinus membrane perforation with a diameter of between 5 and 10 mm, the bone flap from the lateral access window can be used, either in addition to or independently of the use of a resorbable collagen membrane, to perfect the closure of the perforation and facilitate the continuity of the graft. Similarly, in the case of perforations larger than 10 mm in diameter, this bone flap can be used in conjunction with the Bichat fat ball to promote perforation closure.

3.1.5.2. Operating technique [48]

Once the membrane perforation has been identified, further membrane detachment is carried out to reduce stress and allow the membrane to fold back on itself.

The protocol then varies according to the diameter of the perforation:

- For perforations between 5 and 10 mm in diameter:

o The bone flap of the access window is rotated inside the sinus to cover the perforation site.

o A resorbable collagen membrane, larger than the perforation, is applied over the perforation to seal it. The bone flap forming the lateral access window is also rotated inside the sinus to press it against the membrane.

- For perforation diameters greater than 10 mm:
    o The bone flap from the access window is
    rotated inside the sinus to cover the perforation (Figure 31).
  o Next, the fatty Bichat ball is pulled to help close the perforation.

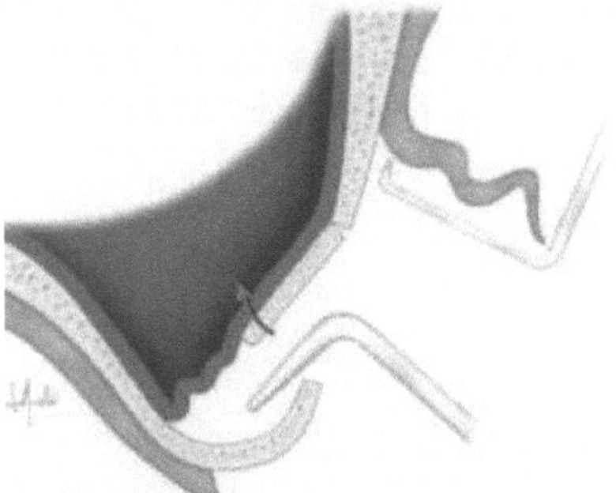

Figure 31: Diagram of the rotation of the bone lamella forming the access window to the interior of the sinus [48].

3.1.6.   Bichat fat ball
3.1.6.1.   Characteristics and anatomy [30,45,109].
The Bichat fat ball, also known as the buccal adipose body, is a pale yellow layer of fat, weighing on average between 8 and 11.5 g, with no significant influence from the patient's age, sex or weight status. Its average dimensions are approximately 10 cm long, 5 cm wide and 2 cm thick. This fat ball consists of a central part, the body, from which extensions emerge.

It is housed in a connective capsule inside the osteo-aponeurotic manducatory cavity, bounded by the buccinator muscle on the medial side and by the masseter and zygomatic arch on the lateral side. It is also important to note that this fat is rich in multipotent cells, thus promoting the healing process of the previously torn membrane.

3.1.6.2.   Indications [45,48]
The Bichat fat ball can be used to obstruct sinus membrane perforations larger than 10 mm in diameter that occur during a lateral approach. The major advantage of this technique lies in the high healing potential of the Bichat fat ball, far surpassing that offered by a conventional collagen membrane.

What's more, this method is relatively simple to use, resistant to infection, does not require vascular anastomosis and offers a degree of comfort for the patient.

3.1.6.3.   Operating technique [45,68]
The Bichat fat ball can be used as a stand-alone method or in conjunction with the application of the bone blade from the access window against the perforation. In either case, the procedure begins by continuing to detach the sinus membrane, with the aim of reducing the tension exerted on it.

The use of the Bichat fat ball initially requires the creation of an approach to access it. This involves a horizontal incision at the base of the vestibule, opposite the second molar. Next, a dissection through the buccinator muscle is made to allow the fat ball to re-enter the oral cavity. The body of the fat ball, together with its extension into the oral cavity, is then gently mobilised for traction to the level of the membrane perforation. A suture at the palatal starting point is then used to position and hold the fat ball in place. Once the perforation has been blocked by the fat ball, the bone substitute material can be introduced and the flap sutured (Figure 32 and 33).

It is important to note that the physiological anatomy of the vestibular fold is restored after approximately 2 months.

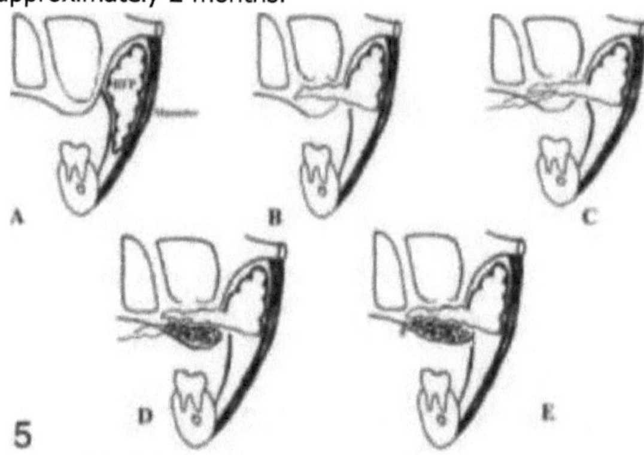

Figure 32: Diagram showing Bic hiat ball traction for obturation of a sinus membrane perforation, with concomitant bone graft [45].

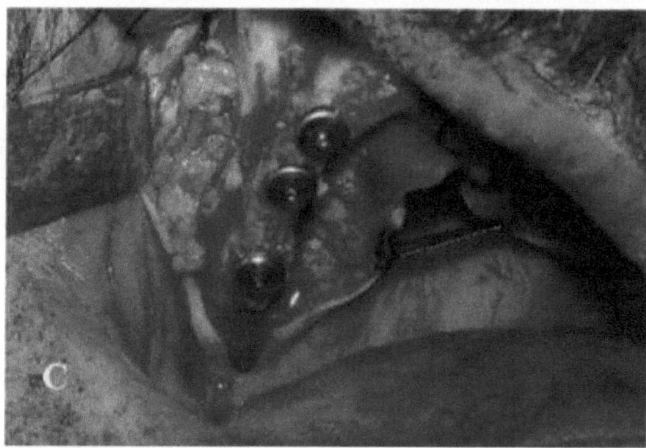

Figure 33: Traction of the Bichat fat ball to the level of the lateral access window [45].

3.1.7. Autogenous or allogeneic bone graft recovery
3.1.7.1. Indications [48,62]

The treatment of sinus membrane perforations larger than 10 mm in diameter can be completed by using an autogenous or allogeneic bone graft in block form. This approach has the advantage of avoiding the usual dispersion of graft material, usually in granular form, within the sinus. In addition, this technique can be used as a stand-alone method or as a complement to another approach to perforation closure.

However, it is important to note that this technique requires a second surgical site if autogenous bone is used. This graft can come either from the iliac crest (which is not discussed here), or from the mandible (symphyseal or retromolar area).

3.1.7.2.   Autogenous graft: harvesting [62,90].

The mandible offers two possible harvesting sites for obtaining an autogenous bone graft suitable for sinus filling:

- **Para-sphysis graft :**

o Advantages: practical surgical access.

o Quantity: Sufficient to treat a gap of two to three teeth.

o Removal: The procedure involves making an osteotomy with a lower limit positioned 3-5 mm from the basilar margin, an upper limit away from the anterior tooth apices, and distal limits that take into account anatomical obstacles such as the inferior alveolar nerve canal and its possible anterior loop.

o Use: The resulting graft can be used to fill the maxillary sinus, and the donor site can be restored with a bone substitute.

- **Mandibular Angle Graft (Ramus or Retromolar Graft)** o Advantages: Provides a larger quantity of bone.

o Harvesting: Carried out at the mandibular angle, it offers a greater quantity of bone. Access requires an osteotomy using a saw-shaped piezoelectric insert and precautions to avoid nerve structures.

o Use: Can be used to fill the maxillary sinus, offering a greater quantity of bone than the paraspyseal graft. The donor site must also be restored.

The choice between these harvesting sites depends on the amount of bone required and the surgeon's preference based on the patient's specific anatomical characteristics.

3.1.7.3.   Operating technique [48,62].

The use of a bone block to cover a sinus membrane perforation generally follows the following steps:

к Continued membrane detachment :

- Objective: To allow the membrane to fold in on itself, thereby limiting the stresses applied.

к Bone sampling :

- If it is an autologous graft, the bone is harvested from the mandible or another suitable source.

к Bone block adaptation :

- The size and shape of the graft (autogenous or allogeneic block) are adjusted to fit the sub-sinus space (Figure 34).

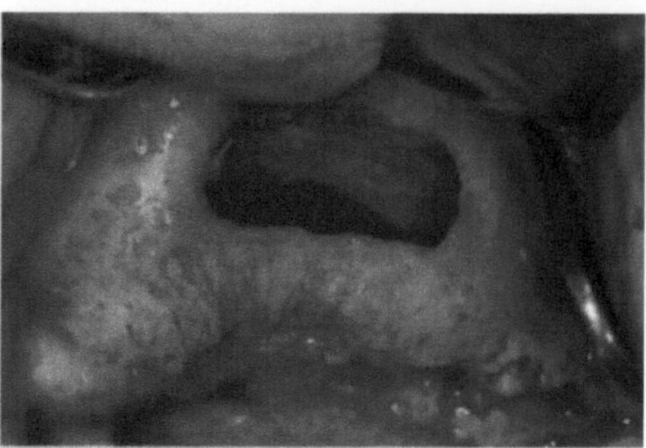

Figure 34: Clinical view of sinus cavity filling with biomaterial [12].

κ Preparation of implant sites :

- The sites where the implants will be placed are prepared using pilot drills.

κ Marking of Implant Sites on the Graft :

- The graft is placed in the sub-sinus space and marked with the future implant sites.

κ Preparation of Implant Sites on the Graft :

- Extra-orally, implant sites are prepared at graft level using conventional drill sequences.

κ Implant placement :

- The implants can be placed in the same surgical procedure, where the implants, once placed, retain the sub-sinus graft. Alternatively, it can be carried out in a second stage, using inter-stage screws.

3.1.8. Closing the perforation with glue

3.1.8.1. Indications [54]

Small sinus membrane perforations, usually less than 5mm in diameter, can be treated with adhesives.

3.1.8.2. Autologous fibrin sealant (figure 35)

κ Biological characteristics [22,95]

The use of autologous fibrin sealant dates back to the first decades of the last century, initially as a hemostatic agent. This substance offers several notable advantages:

1. **Resorption Complete :**

- The fibrin sealant resorbs completely, eliminating the need for secondary interventions.

2. **Autologous and biocompatible :**

- Since it is derived from the patient's own blood, the fibrin sealant is autologous, eliminating any risk of rejection and ensuring perfect biocompatibility.

3. **Ease of use :**

- Handling fibrin sealant is simple and straightforward.

4. **Chemical and physical adhesion :**

- This substance provides both chemical and physical adhesion to fabrics, guaranteeing stability and watertightness.

5. **Hemostasis, bonding and sealing properties:**

- In addition to its hemostatic properties, fibrin sealant has bonding and sealing properties.

6. **Growth Factors :**

- Because of its high platelet concentration, fibrin sealant promotes membrane healing.

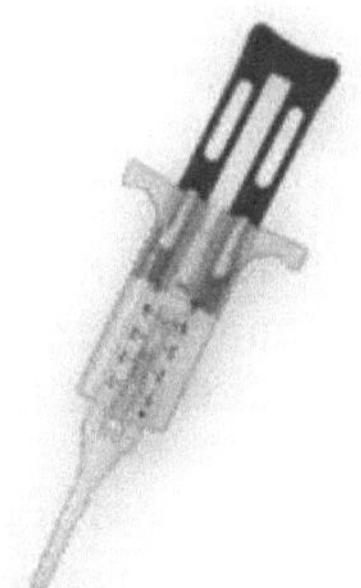

Figure 35: Fibrin sealant [114].

κ Operating technique [22,63]

The use of fibrin sealant to repair a sinus membrane perforation begins by continuing to detach the membrane as soon as the perforation is detected. This step is designed to minimise stress on the membrane. The edges of the perforated membrane are carefully brought together, and the glue is applied with a syringe directly to the perforation.

The position is then held for 60 seconds, allowing the adhesive to set at body temperature. Filling with a bone substitute can then be performed, either directly or after application of the bone flap from the access window to the perforation site.

It should be noted that autologous fibrin sealant can also be used in addition to another means of treating the perforation, such as the application of a Surgicel® membrane. In this situation, the membrane is first applied at the level of the perforation, and then the fibrin sealant is positioned all around the membrane to ensure its stability.

3.1.8.3. Biological glue

κ Biological characteristics [97]

Biological glues, in particular Tissucol® and Beriplast®, are commercial preparations obtained by fractionation of human plasma, with the status of Blood Derived Medicinal Product. They are used in liquid form for the treatment of sinus membrane perforations. Composed of human fibrinogen, human factor XIII, human fibronectin, human thrombin and bovine aprotinin, these components are mixed extemporaneously at the time of application, thereby activating instant coagulation of the constituents. A notable advantage of these adhesives is that they are resorbed within two weeks.

к **Operating technique [22,95]**

The operating procedure for the use of biological glue is similar to that for autologous fibrin glue, comprising the following steps:
- Membrane detachment around the perforation,
- Bringing the edges of the perforation closer together,
- Apply glue to the perforation,
- Hold position for 60 seconds.

In the same way as fibrin sealant, biological sealant can be used independently or in conjunction with another technique for treating sinus membrane perforations.

3.1.9. Resorbable haemostatic

3.1.9.1. Composition [63,93]

Resorbable hemostatic agents such as Surgicel® come in the form of sterile, resorbable compresses. Derived from plant sources, they contain regenerated oxidised cellulose, demonstrating both osteogenic and osteoconductive potential.

3.1.9.2. Indications [93,116]

A resorbable hemostatic membrane can be used to seal sinus membrane perforations larger than 5 mm in diameter. This method has the advantage of being simple, fast, reliable and cost-effective. In addition, unlike fibrin sealants, resorbable hemostatics are ready-to-use and can be stored at room temperature.

3.1.9.3. Operating technique [63,93]

The incorporation of a resorbable hemostatic membrane in the treatment of a sinus membrane perforation always begins with the continued detachment of this membrane, with the aim of reducing the tensions present in it. A hemostatic membrane is then cut to the appropriate size (at least 3 mm larger than the initial perforation) and positioned against the sinus membrane.

By absorbing blood, this hemostatic membrane acquires a gelatinous consistency, giving it mechanical strength and hermetic properties. A delicate Valsava manoeuvre can be performed to check that the seal is complete. If the seal is not complete, a second membrane can be added. The bone substitute can then be inserted in the conventional way. It is important to note that the application of this hemostatic membrane can eventually be completed by the use of fibrin glue or biological glue to perfect the seal.

3.1.10. Palatal connective tissue graft

3.1.10.1. Indications

Palatal connective tissue, commonly used in periodontal surgery, is emerging as a graft source that can also be exploited in the treatment of sinus membrane perforations. Palatal connective tissue offers the advantage of easy access and excellent biological properties. This approach can be considered for the treatment of sinus membrane perforations with a diameter of between 5 and 10 mm.

3.1.10.2. Operating technique [40]

Treatment of sinus membrane perforation begins with detachment of the membrane on either side of the initial perforation in order to reduce the tension exerted on it. Next, a palatal connective tissue graft, slightly larger than the perforation, is harvested following the incisions made for the lateral approach. This procedure involves dissecting the epithelial flap using a 15C blade, in a horizontal direction parallel to the surface of the flap. The resulting graft is placed at the perforation, followed by grafting. Finally, the flap is sutured to complete the treatment. (Figure 36)

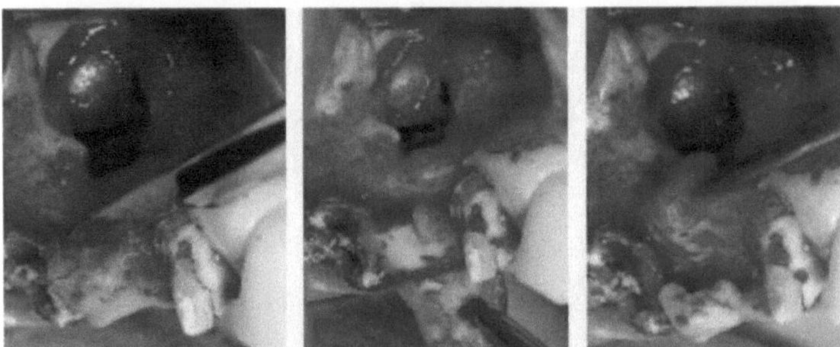

Figure 36: Removal of a palatal connective tissue graft to treat sinus membrane perforation [40].

3.1.11.   Collagen membrane stabilisёe "Loma Linda" technique
3.1.11.1.   Indications [100]
The technique using a stabilised collagen membrane can be used to treat large sinus membrane perforations exceeding 10 mm in diameter.
3.1.11.2.   Benefits [100]
The use of a stabilised collagen membrane in the treatment of sinus membrane perforations is designed to prevent displacement of the collagen membrane during insertion of the bone substitute.

The pocket method, also known as the Loma Linda technique, offers the possibility of performing a lateral bone graft even in the presence of a sinus membrane perforation, by isolating the substitute biomaterial. This method involves placing a resorbable collagen membrane inside the sinus, fixed on either side of the lateral access window with screw anchors. This pocket is then closed at the level of the access window by a second membrane. It is essential to stress that this specific technique has the disadvantage of restricting the vascularisation of the graft, which is completely isolated by the collagen membranes. As a result, there is a delay in the bone remodelling process compared with a conventional graft. (Figure 37, 38)

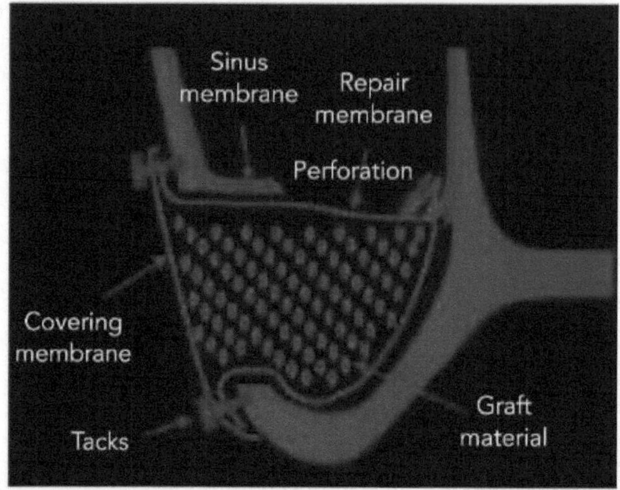

Figure 37: Schematic representation of the Loma Linda technique [83].

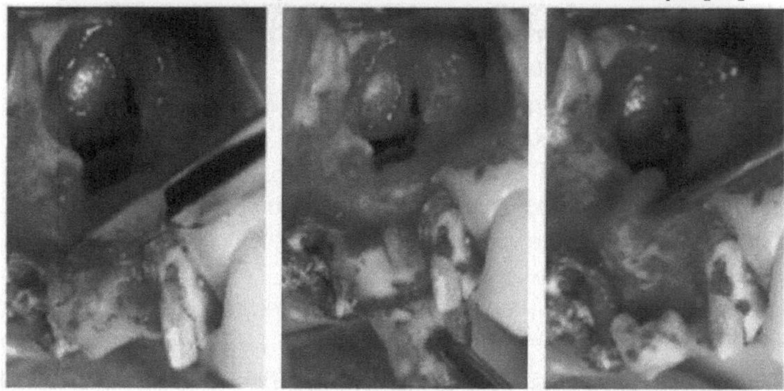

Figure 38: Clinical use of the pouch techn ique, followed by bone substitute placement [83].

3.2. Recommendations, post-operative monitoring and prescription

Following sinus membrane perforation, it is crucial to give the patient appropriate post-operative instructions, in addition to the usual guidelines [48,60]. Here are some specific recommendations:

- Avoid any Valsalva manoeuvre likely to facilitate the passage of sinus secretions through the graft, in order to prevent any risk of graft infection, for one week.
- Refrain from blowing your nose for a week.
- Sneeze with your mouth open for a week after surgery to avoid any overpressure on the sinuses.
- Do not use a straw for vacuuming.
- Avoid flying for a week after the operation.
- Strict adherence to medication prescriptions.

42

An initial post-operative follow-up will be carried out after one week, during which the sutures will be removed. Follow-up consultations will then take place at two weeks, one month and four months after the operation.

The AFFSAPS (Agence fran^aise de securite sanitaire des produits de sante) recommends prophylactic antibiotic treatment for sinus floor elevations in healthy patients [111], in particular :

- 2g Amoxicillin 1 hour before the procedure.

- In case of allergy to penicillins: 600mg of Clindamycin 1 hour before the procedure. Antibiotic prophylaxis should be maintained for seven days in the event of sinus membrane perforation during pre-implant surgery. Some authors, including Antoun [4], recommend a combination of Amoxicillin + Clavulanic Acid 500 mg/62.5 mg twice a day for 7 days (in case of allergy to penicillins: pristinamycin 500 mg twice a day for 7 days), accompanied by prednisolone at a dose of 60 mg the morning after the operation, then 40 mg the morning after.

The post-operative prescription should also include oral level 1 or 2 analgesics (Paracetamol 1 g every 6 hours or Paracetamol codeine 500 mg/30 mg every 6 hours) and mouthwashes with 0.12% Chlorhexidine digluconate (3 times a day for 2 weeks, starting 24 hours after the operation).

Some authors, such as Khitab [61], also suggest the use of a nasal decongestant to alleviate nasal congestion, usually using vasoconstrictors such as ephedrine.

Conclusion

sinus lift. These perforations can occur despite the precautions taken and can compromise the success of the operation.

However, with technological and surgical advances, several techniques are now available to repair these perforations and ensure the bone regeneration required for dental implants.

Small perforations can often be managed using suturing techniques, resorbable collagen membranes or fibrin-based adhesives. These approaches effectively seal the perforation and promote uncomplicated healing.

For larger perforations, various methods of reconstructing the sub-sinus roof have been proposed, including the use of autogenous bone flaps or bone blocks. These techniques offer a reliable solution for restoring the bone roof and allowing bone regeneration.

It is essential that the surgeon is well prepared to manage any perforation that may occur, by having a thorough knowledge of the anatomy of the maxillary sinus and using appropriate techniques. In addition, a full pre-operative assessment, including detailed radiological examinations, is crucial to anticipate any potential complications and choose the best surgical approach for each case.

In conclusion, the management of perforations during sinus lift is an essential element in ensuring the success of sub-sinus bone augmentation and dental implant placement. With a methodical approach, advanced surgical techniques and good pre-operative planning, perforations can be successfully managed, minimising the risk of post-operative complications and ensuring satisfactory results for patients.

Bibliography

1. Abdel-Wahed NA, Bahammam MA. Cone Beam CT-Based Preoperative Volumetric Estimation of Bone Graft Required for Lateral Window Sinus Augmentation, Compared with Intraoperative Findings: A Pilot Study. Open Dent J 2018; 12: 820-6.

2. AFFSAPS. Recommendations for the oral and dental care of patients treated with bisphosphonates. 2007.

3. Al-Faraje L. Risks and complications in implant surgery; Etiology, prevention and management. Paris: Quintessence International; 2012.

4. Antoun H. Les greffes de sinus en implantologie. Paris: Editions CdP, 2020.

5. Arshad A, Patton D, El-Sharkawi AMM. Implant rehabilitation of irradiated jaws: a preliminary report. Inter J Oral Maxillofacial Implants 1997; 12: 523-6.

6. Balaji SM. Direct Vs indirect sinus lift in maxillary dental implants. Ann Maxillofacial Surg 2013; 3: 148-53.

7. Baumann A, Ewers R. Minimal invasive sinus lift. Grenzen und Moglichkeiten im atrophen Oberkiefer. Mund- Kiefer-Gesichtschirurgie MKG 1999; 3 Suppl 1: S70-3.

8. Baykul T, Findik Y. Maxillary sinus perforation with presence of an antral pseudocyst, repaired with platelet rich fibrin. Ann Maxillofac Surg 2014; 4(2): 205-7.

9. Bayol JC, Hardy C, Sury F. Les petits moyens en chirurgie preimplantaire. Rev Stomatol ChirMaxillofac 2009; 110(1): 34-41.

10. Beck-Broichsitter B, Westhoff D, Behrens E, Wiltfang J, Becker S. Impact of surgical management in cases of intraoperative membrane perforation during a sinus lift procedure: a follow-up on bone graft stability and implant success. Int J Implant Dent 2018; 4(1): 6.

11. Becker ST, Terheyden H, Steinriede A, Behrens E, Springer I, Wiltfang J. Prospective observation of 41 perforations of the Schneiderian membrane during sinus floor elevation. Clin Oral Implant Res 2008; 19: 1285-9.

12. Besnier R. Gestion et prevention des complications peroperatoires et post-operatoires des sinus-lift. [These]. Nantes: Unite de formation et de recherche d'odontologie, 2012.

13. Borie E, Olivi DG, Orsi IA, Garlet K, Weber B, Beltran V et al. Platelet-rich fibrin application in dentistry: a literature review. Int J Clin Exp Med 2015; 8(5): 7922-9.

14. Bornstein MM, Seiffert C, Maestre-Ferrin L, Fodich I, Jacobs R, Buser D et al. An Analysis of Frequency, Morphology, and Locations of Maxillary Sinus Septa Using Cone Beam Computed Tomography. Int J Oral Maxillofac Implant 2016; 31: 280-7.

15. Boyne PJ, Lilly LC, Marx RE, Moy PK, Nevins M, Spagnoli DB et al. De novo bone induction by recombinant human bone morphogenetic protein-2 (rhbmp-2) in maxillary sinus floor augmentation. J Oral Maxillofacial Surg 2005; 63(12): 1693-707.

16. Caldwell GW. Diseases of the accessory sinuses of the nose and an improved method of treatment of suppuration of the maxillary antrum. New J Med J 1893; 58: 526-8.

17. **Cavezian R, Pasquet G.** Imagerie dento-maxillaire. Approche radio-clinique. Paris: Masson, 2006.

18. **Chan HL, Suarez F, Monje A, Benavides E, Wang HL.** Evaluation of maxillary sinus width on cone-beam computed tomography for sinus augmentation and new sinus classification based on sinus width. Clin Oral Implant Res 2012; 25: 647-52.

19. **Chen L, Cha J, Chen, Hsin-Chen, Lin HL.** Sinus perforation: treatment and classifications. J Implant Adv Clin Dent 2011; 3(1): 19-30.

20. **Chiapasco M, Felisati G, Maccari A, Borloni R, Gatti F, Di Leo F.** The management of complications following displacement of oral implants in the paranasal sinuses: a multicenter clinical report and proposed treatment protocols. Int J Oral Maxillofac Surg 2009; 38(12): 1273-8.

21. **Cho SC, Wallace SS, Froum SJ, Tarnow DP.** Influence of anatomy on Schneiderian membrane perforations during sinus elevation surgery: three-dimensional analysis. Pract Proced Aesthetic Dent PPAD 2001; 13(2): 160-3.

22. **Choi BH, Zhu SJ, Jung JH, Lee SH, Huh JY.** The use of autologous fibrin glue for closing sinus membrane perforations during sinus lifts. Oral Surg Oral Med Oral Pathol Oral Radiol Endodontology 2006; 101(2): 150-4.

23. **Clementini M, Otttria L, Pandolfi C, Bollero P.** A novel technique to close large perforation of sinus membrane. Oral Implantol 2013; 6(1): 11-4.

24. **Costes V, Sudaka A, Wassef M.** Nasal cavity and sinus polyps: true and false tumours. Ann Pathol 2011; 31(5): S87-91.

25. **Dargaud J, Lamotte C, Dainotti JP, Morin A.** Venous drainage and innervation of the maxillary sinus. Morphologie: Bulletin de I'Association des Anatomistes 2001; 85(270): 1-13.

26. **Davarpanah M, Szmukler-Moncler S.** Simplification of sinus grafts. Paris: Quintessence international, 2011.

27. **Delmas J, Radulesco T, Varoquaux A, Thomassin JM, Dessi P, Michel J.** Anatomy of nasosinus cavities. EMC - Otolaryngology, 2018, 20-265- A-10.

28. **Demurashvili G, Davarpanah K, Rajzbaum Ph.** Manual of clinical implantology: concepts, integration of protocols and outline of new paradigms. 3rd ed. Rueil Malmaison: Editions CdP; 2012.

29. **Ducommun J, Bornstein MM, Wong MCM, von Arx T.** Distances of root apices to adjacent anatomical structures in the anterior maxilla: An analysis using cone beam computed tomography. Clin Oral Investig 2019; 23: 2253-63.

30. **Dumont T, Simon E, Stricker M, Kahn J-L, Chassagne J-F.** La graisse de la face: anatomie descriptive et fonctionnelle partir d'une revue de la litterature et de dissections de dix hemifaces. Ann Chir Plast Esthet 2007; 52(1): 51-61.

31. **Eid J, Abitbol J.** Lateral maxillary sinus grafting associated with implant placement. A class I case. Rev Odont Stomat 2016; 45: 4-20.

32. **Ellaa B, Da Costa Noblea R, Lauverjata Y, Sedarata C, Zwetyengac N,**

Siberchitotc F et al. Septa within the sinus: effect on elevation of the sinus floor. Br J Oral Maxillofac Surg. 2008; 46(6):464-7.

33. **Eloy P, Nollevaux MC, Bertrand B.** Physiology of the paranasal sinuses. EMC-Otolaryngology, 2006, 1(1), 1-10.

34. **Emmerich D, Att W, Stappert C.** Sinus floor elevation using osteotomes: a systematic review and meta- analysis. J Periodontol 2005; 76(8): 1237-51.

35. **Ferreira C, Matinelli C, Novaes-Jr A, Pignaton T.** Effect of maxillary sinus membrane perforation on implant survival rate: a retrospective study. Int J Oral Maxillofac Implants 2017; 32(2): 401-7.

36. **Froum S, Khouly I, Favero G, Cho S.** Effect of maxillary sinus membrane perforation on vital bone formation and implant survival: a retrospective study. J Periodontol 2013; 84(8): 1094-9.

37. **Fugazzotto PA, Vlassis J.** A simplified classification and repair system for sinus membrane perforations. J Periodontol 2003; 74(10): 1534-41.

38. **Galindo P, Sanchez-Fernandez E, Avila G, Cutando A, Fernandez JE.** Migration of implants into the maxillary sinus: two clinical cases. Int J Oral Maxillofac Implants 2005; 20(2): 291-5.

39. **Galindo-Moreno P, Padial-Molina M, Avila G, Rios HF, Hernandez-Cortes P, Wang HL.** Complications associated with implant migration into the maxillary sinus cavity. Clin Oral Implants Res 2012; 23(10): 1152-60.

40. **Gehrke SA, Taschieri S, Del Fabbro M, Corbella S.** Repair of a Perforated Sinus Membrane with a Subepithelial Palatal Conjunctive Flap: Technique Report and Evaluation. Int J Dent 2012; 2012: 1-7.

41. **Gonzalez-Santana H, Penarrocha-Diago M, Guarinos-Carbo J, Sorni-Broker M.** A Study of the Septa in the Maxillary Sinuses and the Subantral Alveolar Processes in 30 Patients. J Oral Implantol 2007; 33(6): 340-3.

42. **Gosau M, Rink D, Driemel O, Draenert F.** Maxillary Sinus Anatomy: A Cadaveric Study With Clinical Implications. Anat Rec Adv Integr Anat Evol Biol 2009; 292(3): 352-4.

43. **Gouët E, Toure G.** Sinus & implant: sinus elevation surgery a visee implantaire. Malakoff: Editions CdP; 2017.

44. **Greenstein G, Cavallaro J, Tarnow D.** Practical application of anatomy for the dental implant surgeon. J Periodontol 2008; 79: 1833-46.

45. **Hassani A, Khojasteh A, Alikhasi M.** Repair of the Perforated Sinus Membrane with Buccal Fat Pad During Sinus Augmentation. J Oral Implantol 2008; 34(6): 330-3.

46. **Hauret L, Hodez C.** Novelty in dento-maxillofacial radiology: cone-beam volumetric tomography. J Radiol 2009; 90: 604-17.

47. **Haute Autorite de Sante.** Prophylaxis of infective endocarditis. Revision de la conference de consensus de mars 1992. Medecine et Maladies Infectieuses 2002; 32: 533-41.

48. **Hernandez-Alfaro F, Torradeflot MM, Marti C.** Prevalence and management of Schneiderian membrane perforations during sinus-lift procedures. Clin Oral Impl

Res 2008; 19: 91-8.

49. Jacobs R, Scarfe WC. Dental Implants. In: Scarfe WC, Angelopoulos C. Maxillofacial Cone Beam Computed Tomography: Principles, Techniques and Clinical Applications. Cham, Switzerland : Eds. Springer International Publishing, 2018; pp. 745-830.

50. Jankowski R, Nguyen DT, Poussel M, Chenuel B, Gallet P, Rumeau C. Sinusology. Ann Fr Oto-rhino-laryngol Pathol Cervico-facial 2016; 133(4): 237-43.

51. Janner SF, Caversaccio MD, Dubach P, Sendi P, Buser D, Bornstein MM. Characteristics and dimensions of the Schneiderian membrane: A radiographic analysis using cone beam computed tomography in patients referred for dental implant surgery in the posterior maxilla. Clin Oral Implant Res 2011; 22: 1446-53.

52. Janner SFM, Dubach P, Suter VGA, Caversaccio MD, Buser D, Bornstein MM. Sinus floor elevation or referral for further diagnosis and therapy: A comparison of maxillary sinus assessment by ENT specialists and dentists using cone beam computed tomography. Clin Oral Implant Res 2020; 31: 463-75.

53. Jensen OT, Shulmanl B, Block MS, Iacono VJ. Report of the sinus consensus conference of 1996. Int J Oral Maxillofac Implants 1998; 13: 11-45.

54. Johan PA, Christiaan M, Disch FJM, Tuinzing DB. Anatomical aspects of sinus floor elevations. Clin Oral Implants Res 2000; 11(3): 256-65.

55. Joung WJ, Yun SH, Kim Y, Cho YS, Lee WW, Seo JW. Intra-sinus rigid fixation of a resorbable barrier membrane to repair a large perforation of the sinus membrane: a technical note. J Korean Assoc Oral Maxillofac Surg 2023; 49(5): 297-303.

56. Kahnberg KE, Wallstrom M, Rasmusson L. Local sinus lift for single-tooth implant. I. clinical and radiographic follow-up. Clin Implant Dent Relat Res 2011; 13: 231-7.

57. Kan JYK, Rungcharassaeng K, Kim J, Lozada JL, Goodacre CJ. Factors affecting the survival of implants placed in grafted maxillary sinuses: a clinical report. J Prosthet Dent 2002; 87(5): 485-9.

58. Kang SJ, Shin SI, Herr Y, Kwon YH, Kim GT, Chung JH. Anatomical structures in the maxillary sinus related to lateral sinus elevation: a cone beam computed tomographic analysis. Clin Oral Implants Res 2013; 24: 75-81.

59. Kao DWK. Clinical Maxillary Sinus Elevation Surgery. Ed. John Wiley & Sons, Inc, 2014.

60. Katsuyama H, Jensen SS. ITI Treatment Guide. Volume 5: Les procedures d'elevation du plancher du sinus. Paris: Quintessence Publishing, 2012.

61. Khitab U, Khan A, Khan MT, Shah SMA. Treatment of Oroantral Fistula-a Study. Pak Oral Dent J 2010; 30(2): 27-30.

62. Khoury F. Augmentation of the Sinus Floor with Mandibular Bone Block and Simultaneous Implantation: A 6-Year Clinical Investigation. Int J Oral Maxillofac Implants 1999; 14(4): 557-64.

63. Kim YK, Choe GY, Yun PY. Management of Perforated Sinus Membrane Using Absorbable Haemostat and Fibrin Adhesive for Sinus Lift Procedure. Asian J Oral

Maxillofac Surg 2008; 20(3): 129-34.

64. Kluppel LE, Santos SE, Olate S, Freire Filho FWV, Moreira RWF, de Moraes M. Implant migration into maxillary sinus: description of two asymptomatic cases. Oral Maxillofac Surg 2010; 14(1): 63-6.

65. Langer B, Langer L. Use of allograft for sinus grafting. In: The sinus bone graft. Chicago: Quintessence Publishing, 1999. 69-78.

66. Lee WJ, Lee SJ, Kim HS. Analysis of location and prevalence of maxillary sinus septa. J Periodontal Implant Sci 2010; 40(2): 56-60.

67. Lim EL, Ngeow WC, Lim D. The implications of different lateral wall thicknesses on surgical access to the maxillary sinus. Braz Oral Res 2017; 31: e97.

68. Liversedge RL, Wong K. Use of the Buccal Fat Pad in Maxillary and Sinus Grafting of the Severely Atrophic Maxilla Preparatory to Implant Reconstruction of the Partially or Completely Edentulous Patient: Technical Note. Int J Oral Maxillofac Implants 2002; 17(3): 424-8.

69. Luc H. A new operative method for the radical cure of chronic empyema of the maxillary sinus. Arch Inter Laryngol Otologie Rhinologie 1897; 10: 273-85.

70. Massei G, Romano F, Aimetti M. An Innovative Technique to Manage Sinus Membrane Perforations: Report of Two Cases. Int J Periodontics Restorative Dent 2015; 35(3): 372-9.

71. Meleo D, Mangione F, Corbi S, Pacifici L. Management of the Schneiderian membrane perforation during the maxillary sinus elevation procedure: a case report. Ann Stomatol (Roma) 2012; 3(1): 24-30.

72. Misch CE, Judy KW. Classification of partially edentulous arches for implant dentistry. Int J Oral Implantol Implantol 1987; 4(2): 7-13.

73. Monje A, Diaz KT, Aranda L, Insua A, Garcia-Nogales A, Wang HL. Schneiderian Membrane Thickness and Clinical Implications for Sinus Augmentation: A Systematic Review and Meta-Regression Analyses. J Periodontol 2016; 87: 888-99.

74. Neugebauer J, Ritter L, Mischkowski RA, Dreiseidler T, Scherer P, Ketterle M et al. Evaluation of maxillary sinus anatomy by cone-beam CT prior to sinus floor elevation. Int J Oral Maxillofac Implant 2010; 25: 258-65.

75. Oh E, Kraut E. Effect of sinus membrane perforation on dental implant integration: a retrospective study on 128 patients. Implant Dent 2011; 20(1): 13-9.

76. Oncu E, Kaymaz E. Assessment of the effectiveness of platelet rich fibrin in the treatment of Schneiderian membrane perforation. Clin Implant Dent Relat Res 2017; 19(6): 1009-14.

77. Park WB, Han J, Kang P, Momen-Heravi F. The clinical and radiographic outcomes of Schneiderian membrane perforation without repair in sinus elevation surgery. Clin Implant Dent Relat Res 2019; 21(5): 931-7.

78. Pasquet G, Cavezian R. Diagnostic means in odonto- stomatological cone beam imaging: results. J Radiol 2009; 90: 618-23.

79. Perros N. Schneider's membrane perforations in sinus fillers: Prevention and management of complications. [These]. Lorraine : Faculte d'Odontologie, 2016.

80. Pommer B, Ulm C, Lorenzoni M, Palmer R, Watzek G, Zechner W.

Prevalence, location and morphology of maxillary sinus septa: systematic review and meta-analysis. J Clin Periodontol 2012; 39(8): 769-73.

81. **Princ G, Piral T.** Preimplant bone surgery. Paris: Editions CdP, 2008.

82. **Proussaefs P, Lozada J, Kim J, Rohrer MD.** Repair of the Perforated Sinus Membrane with a Resorbable Collagen Membrane: A Human Study. Int J Oral Maxillofac Implants 2004; 19(3): 413-20.

83. **Proussaefs P, Lozada J.** The "Loma Linda Pouch": A Technique for Repairing the Perforated Sinus Membrane. Int J Periodontics Restorative Dent 2003; 23(6): 592-7.

84. **Rahpeyma A, Khajehahmadi S.** Open Sinus Lift Surgery and the Importance of Preoperative Cone-Beam Computed Tomography Scan: A Review. J Int Oral Health 2015; 7: 127-33.

85. **Robiony M, Tenani G, Sbuelz M, Casadei M.** A simple method for repairing membrane sinus perforation. Open J Stomatol 2012; 2: 348-51.

86. **Rosano G, Gaudy JF, Chaumanet G, Del Fabbro M, Taschieri S.** Maxillary sinus septa. Prevalence and anatomy through a review of the literature from 1980 to 2009. Rev Stomatol Chir Maxillofac 2012; 113(1): 32-5.

87. **Scarano A, Murmura G, Mastrangelo F, Lorusso F, Lucchina AG, Carinci F.** A novel technique to prevent sinus membrane collapse during maxillary sinus floor augmentation without bone graft: technical note. Journal of Biological Regulators and Homeostatic Agents 2018; 32(6):1589-92.

88. **Schlegel AK, Mohler H, Busch F, Mehl A.** Preclinical and clinical studies of a collagen membrane (Bio-Gide®). Biomaterials 1997; 18(7): 535-8.

89. **Schriber M, Von Arx T, Sendi P, Jacobs R, Suter VG, Bornstein MM.** Evaluating Maxillary Sinus Septa Using Cone Beam Computed Tomography: Is There a Difference in Frequency and Type Between the Dentate and Edentulous Posterior Maxilla? Int J Oral Maxillofac Implant 2017; 32: 1324-32.

90. **Seban A, Bonnaud P.** Clinical practice of bone grafts and implants. Modalites therapeutiques et prise en charge des complications. Issy-Les Moulineaux: Elsevier Masson, 2012.

91. **Seban A.** Bone grafts and implants. Issy-les-moulineaux: Elsevier Masson; 2008.

92. **Shanbhag S, Karnik P, Shirke P, Shanbhag V.** Cone-beam computed tomographic analysis of sinus membrane thickness, ostium patency, and residual ridge heights in the posterior maxilla: Implications for sinus floor elevation. Clin Oral Implant Res 2013; 25: 755-60.

93. **Simunek A, Kopecka D, Cierny M.** The Use of Oxidized Regenerated Cellulose (Surgicel®) in closing Schneiderian Membrane Tears during the Sinus Lift Procedure. West Indian Med J 2005; 54(6): 398-9.

94. **Stricker M, Raphael B, Gerard H, Dambrain R.** Croissance cranio faciale: Normale et pathologique, I'interception therapeutique et son devenir. Reims, France: Ed. Morfos, 1993.

95. **Sullivan SM, Bulard RA, Meaders R, Patterson MK.** The use of fibrin adhesive in sinus lift procedures. Oral Surg Oral Med Oral Pathol Oral Radiol

Endodontology 1997; 84(6): 616-9.

96. **Summers RB.** A new concept in maxillary implant surgery: the osteotome technique. Compendium of Continuing Education in Dentistry 1994; 2: 152-60.

97. **Summers RB.** Sinus floor elevation with osteotomes. J Esthet Dent 1998; 10(3): 164-71.

98. **Tatum H.** Maxillary and sinus implant reconstruction. Dental Clinics of North America 1986; 30: 227-9.

99. **Tavelli L, Borgonovo AE, Re D, Maiorana C.** Sinus presurgical evaluation: A literature review and a new classification proposal. Minerva Stomatol 2017; 66: 115-31.

100. **Testori T, Wallace SS, Del Fabbro M, Taschieri S, Trisi P, Capelli M et al.** Repair of Large Sinus Membrane Perforations Using Stabilized Collagen Barrier Membranes: Surgical Techniques with Histologic and Radiographic Evidence of Success. Int J Periodontics Restorative Dent 2008; 28(1): 8-17.

101. **Tsodoulos S, Karabouta I, Voulgaropoulou M, Georgiou C.** Atraumatic Removal of an Asymptomatic Migrated Dental Implant into the Maxillary Sinus: A Case Report. J Oral Implantol 2012; 38(2): 189-93.

102. **Tyndall DA, Price JB, Tetradis S, Ganz SD, Hildebolt C, Scarfe WC.** Position statement of the American Academy of Oral and Maxillofacial Radiology on selection criteria for the use of radiology in dental implantology with emphasis on cone beam computed tomography. Oral Surg Oral Med Oral Pathol Oral Radiol 2012; 113: 817-26.

103. **Van den Bergh JP, ten Bruggenkate CM, Disch FJ, Tuinzing DB.** Anatomical aspects of sinus floor elevations. Clin Oral Implants Res 2000; 11(3): 256-65.

104. **Velasquez-Plata D, Hovey LR, Peach CC, Alder ME.** Maxillary sinus septa: a 3-dimensional computerized tomographic scan analysis. Int J Oral Maxillofac Implants 2002; 17(6): 854-60.

105. **Von Arx T, Fodich I, Bornstein MM, Jensen SS.** Perforation of the Sinus Membrane During Sinus Floor Elevation: A Retrospective Study of Frequency and Possible Risk Factors. Int J Oral Maxillofac Implants 2014; 29(3): 718-26.

106. **Wen SC, Chan HL, Wang HL.** Classification and management of antral septa for maxillary sinus augmentation. Int J Periodontics Restorative Dent 2013; 33(4): 50917.

107. **Yeung AWK, Colsoul N, Montalvao C, Hung K, Jacobs R, Bornstein MM.** Visibility, location, and morphology of the primary maxillary sinus ostium and presence of accessory ostia: A retrospective analysis using cone beam computed tomography (CBCT). Clin Oral Investig 2019; 23: 3977-86.

108. **Young B, O'Dowd G, Woodford P.** Wheater's functional histology: A text and colour atlas (Sixth edition). Philadelphia, PA: Churchill Livingston/Elsevier, 2014.

109. **Young-Kyun K, Jung-Won H, Pil-Young Y.** Closure of Large Perforation of Sinus Membrane Using Pedicled Buccal Fat Pad Graft: A Case Report. Int J Oral Maxillofac Implants 2008; 23(6): 1139-42.

110. Zijderveld SA, van den Bergh JP, Schulten EA, ten Bruggenkate CM. Anatomical and surgical findings and complications in 100 consecutive maxillary sinus floor elevation procedures. J Oral Maxillofac Surg 2008; 66: 1426-38.

Internet references

111. French Health Products Safety Agency (AFSSAPS). Recommendations July 2011: Prescription of antibiotics in oral and dental practice. [On line]. 2011 [consulted on 14/08/2023]. Available from: http://ansm.sante.fr/Dossiers/Antibiotiques/Odonto-Stomatology/(offset)/ 5

112. Baron Dental Clinic. Bone Grafting in Turkey. [Online]. 2023 [Accessed 5/11/2023]. Available at: https://www.sidedentalclinic.com/en/treatment/7/ bone-grafting-in-turkey

113. Bauer B. Sinus lift. [Online]. 2022 [Accessed 25/10/2023]. Available from: https://www.bauersmiles.com/2012/10/sinus-lift.html/

114. Baxter Tisseel Kit Fibrin Sealant-2ml. [Online]. 2023 [Accessed 25/10/2023]. Available from: https://www.hospitalstore.com/baxter-tisseel-kit- fibrin-sealant/

115. Geistlich. Lateral Sinus Floor Elevation. [Online]. 2021 [Accessed on 25/10/2023]. Available from: https://www.geistlich-na.com/dental-professionals/therapeutic-areas/sinus-floor-elevation/lateral-sinus-floor-elevation

116. Haute Autorite de Sante. Rapport d'évaluation technologique sur les Hemostatiques chirurgicaux (HAS). [Online]. 2011 [Accessed 14/08/2023]. Available from: http://www.has-sante.fr/portail/upload/docs/application/pdf/ 2011-07/rapport_hemostatiques_27052011_vd.pdf

117. The nasal cavity and paranasal sinuses. [Online]. 2020 [Accessed 5/11/2023]. Available from: https://doc-pedagogie.umontpellier.fr/medecine/ histologieLV/index.php?module=detail&subaction=desc&vue=4&itm=116&g= 1&d=1

118. Sinus Lift: Definition, Procedures, Cost and Recovery Duration. [On-line]. 2023 [Consultele 5/11/2023]. Available from: https://www.myradental.co.uk/sinus-lift-definition-procedures-cost-and-recovery-duration/

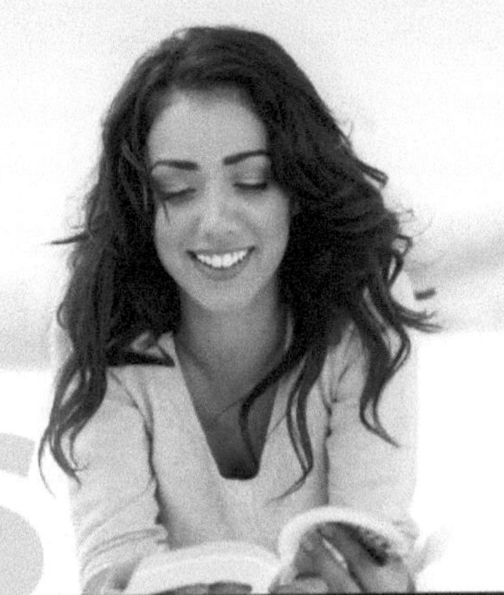

yes
I want morebooks!

Buy your books fast and straightforward online - at one of world's fastest growing online book stores! Environmentally sound due to Print-on-Demand technologies.

Buy your books online at
www.morebooks.shop

Kaufen Sie Ihre Bücher schnell und unkompliziert online – auf einer der am schnellsten wachsenden Buchhandelsplattformen weltweit! Dank Print-On-Demand umwelt- und ressourcenschonend produzi ert.

Bücher schneller online kaufen
www.morebooks.shop

info@omniscriptum.com
www.omniscriptum.com

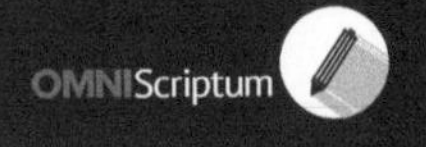

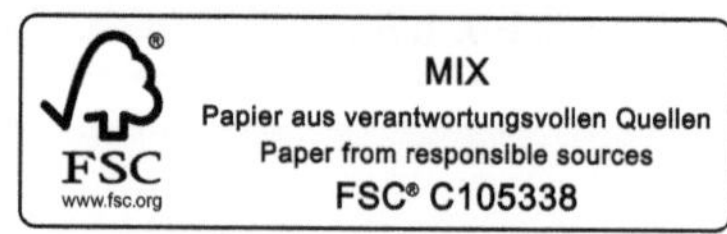